BJJ AFTER 40 SURVIVAL GUIDE MASTERS EDITION

Unlocking the Secrets to Jiu-Jitsu for the Ageless Athlete

By: Mike 'Spider Ninja' Bidwell

Sheena Bidwell

Forward by Michael Musumeci Sr.

*With Contributions from Survival Experts:

Clark Gregg

Brent Burniston

Ryan Ford

Marco Lala

Ari Knazan

Vlad Koulikov

Bong Abad

Marty Josey

Mike Jolly

Mark "Funk" Roberts

Garry Parrett

XMartial

BJJ After 40 Survival Guide Masters Edition
© 2024 by Mike & Sheena Bidwell. All rights reserved.

First Edition

979-8-9907378-0-8 paperback ISBN
979-8-9907378-1-5 Ebook - EPUB ISBN

Published by FLO Life
9191 West Jewell Avenue
BJJAfter40@gmail.com

www.BJJAfter40.com

Cover Design by Mike & Sheena Bidwell
Interior Formatting by Mike & Sheena Bidwell

Distribution by Amazon, Audible, Barnes & Noble and
other digital platforms.

This book is dedicated to Brazilian Jiu-Jitsu.
May this art continue to live, grow and give
within all of us.

Table of Contents

Forward

The human body is a complex machine, the most complex machine on earth, but it has one major flaw… it's inevitably going to break down. This breakdown can have a devastating impact on one's quality of life and mental state.

My name is Michael Musumeci, and a couple of years ago I was experiencing such an issue. I had severe muscle pain and weakness, particularly in the areas I had injured in the past.

Being in my sixties, I was beginning to think my days of any type of physical activity were behind me. After all, I've been active up until then, but there was no doubt my body was beat up. After a physical examination, a multitude of diagnostic tests and extensive blood work, which all came back negative, I was beginning to come to terms with the realization that maybe time caught up with me in a big way. I saw a nutritionist, a physical therapist and even an acupuncturist to no avail. In desperation, I continued to look for answers on the internet.

It was during that time that I came across BJJ After 40 and Mike Bidwell. Mike was a Brazilian Jiu-Jitsu black belt who owned FLO Life, an academy located in Colorado. I wrote him and explained the problems I was having. He wrote me back the same day! I was taken aback by his kindness and willingness to help a stranger. He suggested some supplements he had been using for years. I ordered the supplements he had advised, and they worked!

Both my son and daughter, Mikey and Tammi Musumeci have been competing in Jiu-Jitsu for many years, so I'm no stranger to proper nutrition and supplementation. But Mike's recommendations worked!

Recognizing a lack of resources and a support system for grapplers over 40 and above, Mike took the initiative to bridge the gap. He founded BJJ After 40, a global community-driven platform that offers more than just techniques and training tips, it's a haven for mature BJJ enthusiasts. It fosters connections, sharing stories of resilience, and showcasing that age, in many ways, remains a mere number when passion and determination drive an individual. Through his efforts with BJJ After 40, Mike has been instrumental in challenging age-related stereotypes in the martial arts world. Mike's philosophy does not transcend to just BJJ.

He integrates a holistic approach to his practice, drawing from disciplines like mindfulness meditation. This integrative perspective underscores the idea that BJJ is not just a physical endeavor but a journey of the mind and spirit as well. Mike has often emphasized the importance of staying flexible, not just in body, but in thought and approach, adapting to the ever-evolving journey of life and martial arts.

In addition to being an ambassador for older BJJ practitioners, Mike Bidwell is a beacon of inspiration for all ages, reminding us that with dedication, adaptability, and a love for the journey, any obstacle can be transformed into an opportunity. Mike is a father to four fellow BJJ enthusiasts, and his wife Sheena is also a BJJ black belt.

BJJ After 40 Survival Guide is a must have for those who are aging and want to continue to remain active in their respective sports. This book helps address different issues that those of us who are aging experience and allows the prevention of things before they inevitably will happen.

Understanding the body and the aging process allows for the practitioner to make needed changes to encourage continued success.

Staying active is important as we age, and doing things responsibly will prevent future problems that may slow us down and force us to age more quickly.

Mike has given those of us over 40 a great gift. He provided us with a practical guide to prevent injury and heal from injuries we already have, through needed nutrition and supplementation. This guide will enable us to perform in the best way we can and to be educated on past, present, and future obstacles. BJJ After 40 is a must.

Mike changed my life and helped me to feel better physically, and therefore, mentally. I cannot recommend this book more, and all the knowledge he shares.

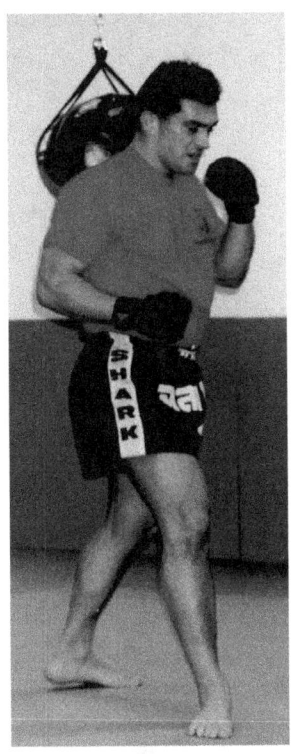

Mike M. Sr.

Introduction

Welcome to the Masters Edition of the BJJ After 40 Survival Guide, where we've engineered a groundbreaking evolution in training. This isn't just a book; it's an interactive experience, bridging the gap between traditional reading and digital engagement. As you navigate through these pages, you'll encounter QR codes. Scan them with your smartphone to unlock a wealth of multimedia content—videos demonstrating techniques, audio guides for meditation, and more, enriching your learning experience with every page turned.

Join us on The BJJ After 40 Survival Guide Masters Edition
YouTube Channel at:

https///www.youtube.com/channel/
UC2zkgjf5RpVPqZjJE6uQ3Tg

As a veteran, I've integrated the disciplined structure of military life into the format of this guide. The book is divided into four strategic sections:

1. Foundations of Jiu-Jitsu Mastery

2. On the Mats

3. Off the Mats

4. Continuing the Journey

Within each section lies a series of "operations," each representing a mission in itself—if you choose to accept them. These missions are designed not just for reading but for deep, active engagement, applying each lesson directly to your BJJ training.

We crafted this guide in the spirit of military precision and strategic focus. Missions in this guide are like those in the military—defined tasks with objectives crucial to your development in BJJ. Every operation concludes with a debriefing, an essential phase where we'll regroup to consolidate what's been learned, identify what's worked, and strategize improvements. This process mirrors the military approach of after-action reviews, critical for ongoing success and adaptation.

Our community's rich collection of experiences and wisdom—from seasoned BJJ black belts to elite fitness coaches and insightful corporate strategists—enriches this edition. They contribute not just knowledge but a shared spirit of resilience and growth.

My own path to a black belt took a unique route, with a significant pause at brown belt before achieving the milestone in 2014. This path instilled in me a profound sense of purpose: to give back and uplift others. As the saying goes, the best time to plant a tree was 20 years ago, and the second-best time is now. By engaging with this guide, you take an active step towards profound personal and community growth.

This guide aims to arm you with more than just techniques; it's here to help you lead a richer, more disciplined life, imbued with the core values of Brazilian Jiu-Jitsu. It is more than a manual; it is a roadmap to resilience, community leadership, and personal fulfillment. Here, every technique learned and every challenge overcome is a step toward building your enduring impact.

Welcome to the BJJ After Forty Masters Edition—your mission begins now. Take on this comprehensive approach to Jiu-Jitsu, where the process is just as important as the results, and every step you take builds the foundation for lasting success and fulfillment.

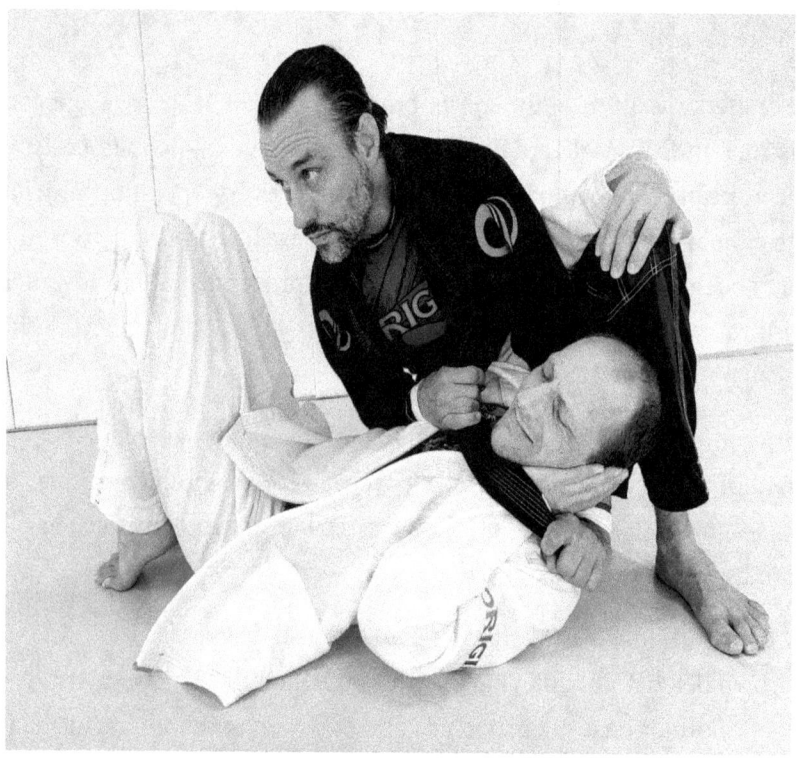

Mike Bidwell

PART I:
FOUNDATIONS OF
JIU-JITSU MASTERY

Operations:
<u>Mental Jiu-Jitsu</u>

Chapters on mental strategies, learning techniques, and overcoming psychological barriers with insights from experts in psychology and top athletes.

Scan the QR code to watch strategies and mental frameworks that enhance your grappling mindset.

https///www.youtube.com/playlist?list=
PLwb5iQup993_-N0vIlzw7BDyntaRtD4QL

Philosophy of Jiu-Jitsu

It's hard to ignore all of the important parallels between Jiu-Jitsu and life. These two align well because both demand evolution, strategic thinking, and a commitment to self control. In BJJ and life we face challenges that require adaptability and improvisation. On the mats we will experience the unrelenting pressure of side control. Through our training we quickly learn that panicking only makes things worse.

We eventually realize that only by accepting our circumstances, can we move forward with a plan. It is in our resistance of the experience that causes us to feel frustration and panic. When you meet resistance with resistance, nobody wins. But if we meet it with a new angle and opportunity we put ourselves on a path to growth and discovery. This shift in perspective allows us to turn blockages into bridges, gifting us a growth mind-set of adaptability and resilience.

The core concept that underscores Jiu-Jitsu is to employ *"minimum effort for maximum results."* This is what allows a much smaller person to defend themselves against a larger opponent. The advantage isn't strength but rather a combination of leverage, timing and the proper execution of a technique. The latter do not require physical prowess. But by adding strength, speed or athleticism to the mix it does create a formidable advantage.

Taking it easy:

By facing our difficulties head on they can often reveal new possibilities and opportunities. Jiu-Jitsu can be translated as the "gentle art." Which can also be further expanded as, "bending or pliable art." As a younger practitioner I didn't fully understand the dichotomy. How could this brutal martial art be considered 'gentle.' I thought, "There's very little *gentle* in Jiu-Jitsu!" It should be noted that the term 'gentle' does *not* imply that Jiu-Jitsu is weak or a passive martial art. The idea of being *gentle* in Jiu-Jitsu can be traced back to the samurai. They recognized the importance of efficiency and energy conservation during warfare. They saw the complexity of combat, the mind-body strategy often tipping the balance between life and death.

The concept of Jiu-Jitsu being pliable and bending extends beyond the physical manifestations, reaching deep into the realm of mental fortitude and resilience. The "bending" in Jiu-Jitsu can be likened to a young sapling of a tree. The small "weak" tree will bend and move with strong winds. Whereas a larger, more "powerful" tree may become a victim to stronger winds.

Just like the smaller tree that sways and moves with the wind, the BJJ practitioner bends with their circumstances and flows with the current of the fight. My first instructional video was called "**Flow-Jitsu.**" The catch phrase was, "**Don't fight the flow. Flow the fight.**" We chose this because it really captures the essence of Jiu-Jitsu and its philosophical approach to combat and life. BJJ emphasizes flexibility, adaptability, and the intelligent conservation of energy. Just as the smaller tree doesn't resist but instead moves with the wind, leveraging its force rather than opposing it directly, a BJJ practitioner learns to work with the momentum and energy of their opponent. They understand that rigid resistance often leads to exhaustion or defeat, while flexibility and adaptability can directly impact the outcome of an encounter (on and off the mats).

What we face on the mats lend to a sense of mental toughness that permeates all aspects of the practitioners life. This in turn allows them to navigate obstacles with focus and composure. Each roll is a test of fortitude and mental suppleness. Through our practice of we learn to manage stress, handle pressure and tolerate discomfort. This ability to stay clam under difficult situations, is often called the practice of "stoicism."

The philosophy of **stoicism** comes from ancient Greece. At its core, it proposes the idea that **we may not be able to control our circumstances, but we can control how we respond to them**. By shifting our perspective and focusing on our reactions versus the events themselves, we can empower ourselves and take hold of the situation.

<u>**Now imagine two grappling scenarios:**</u>

- Number One: You're "stuck" in side control. The pressure from the top feels horrible and there's no escape. You begin to elevate your hips to attempt to bump them off, but to no avail. You try everything and nothing seems to work. You're tired, breathing heavy and out of energy and panic begins to set in. You feel like you're about to die!

- Number Two: Now imagine you're in bottom side control. You're on your back with your partner on top. Your breathing is relaxed and in control. You're aware of your body and limbs in relationship to your partners positioning. Your thoughts are focused and clear. You patiently wait for your partner to make a move so you can consciously counter.

These are the same exact scenarios, but with completely different perspectives.

In number one you're "stuck" in side control, whereas in number two I called it "bottom side control." Where would you rather be?

In the first scenario where it appears that there's no escape and you're suffering in the bowels of hell?

Or would you rather be in situation number two? In this scenario there's no panic. You are not wasting energy on unimportant things. Instead, you're calmly interpreting the situation through focused breathing and a clear, composed mind. You recognize that you're not trapped and there's no need for reckless expenditures of energy. You wait patiently, focused on the subtleties in your partners movements. Every shift in weight, every small movement feeds into your mental map of the situation. This allows you to conserve energy and inform your next move. This is the true mindset of a warrior! You're not giving up, nor are you diving head first into the fray. Instead you're engaged in a delicate dance of strategy and patience. This is how you 'play the game', versus becoming a victim to your opponents strategy.

It is vital to recognize that even in the face of fear that you are not driven by the impulse of uncontrolled aggression. Or just simply giving up.

Let's talk about the core of our art—Philosophy of Jiu-Jitsu. This isn't just about techniques; it's about the approach to life and learning. Philosophy in Jiu-Jitsu integrates concepts like respect, persistence, and mindfulness, and it teaches us the value of patience and resilience. It's not just what we do; it's who we become on and off the mats.

Stay Graced:

You may have heard the phrase, "grace under pressure." The word "**grace**" is interesting because its definition is multifaceted. In the context of physical movement, grace refers to being **smooth and effortless**. In social environments it refers to being **polite and considerate**. In the context of adversity it means to **remain poised and calm under even the most dire circumstances.**

Now let's take a look at the opposite of grace. In the context of physical movements potential antonyms might be: clumsiness, awkward, uncoordinated. In social environments you might think of rudeness or being impolite. For grace in the context of adversity potential antonyms might include: panic, agitation and flustered.

Now you might read that and say, "I'm all those in BJJ: clumsy, awkward, etc." The first step to changing this thought pattern is to acknowledge that it's there. Understanding your own mindset is crucial to your personal growth. You may be awkward at BJJ now, but that won't last forever. Even the most talented Jiu-Jitsu black belt started as an uninformed, "spazzy" beginner. If you see yourself as clumsy today, you're not doomed to remain so.

After all my years teaching BJJ, I have never come across someone who doesn't have a breakthrough. If you stick with it long enough, everyone gets good. The key is a commitment to consistency and continuous learning. Every time you are "clumsy" or get tapped these are opportunities for personal growth. When you "make mistakes" you're just identifying areas of improvement. There's power in that data! You have to be willing to embrace these moments, not as failures, but as stepping stones towards mastery.

A teacher once told me, "feedback is the breakfast of champions!" What he meant was that "feedback," whether it's positive or negative, is vital to personal growth. Let's say for example, you're constantly getting stuck in side control. You may think that you need better side control escapes. Or worse, you might just think you just suck at BJJ and there's nothing that can be done.

But if you dug a little deeper, you might see that you need a better guard game. The reality is that getting in side control was just a consequence of having your guard passed. But if you were unwilling to evaluate your own BJJ game, how could ever find the holes in the bucket? The hole in the bucket story is a metaphorical tale used to explain the concept of futile effort and reoccurring failures that aren't addressed at their root cause.

The story goes like this:

"There was a boy who was given the chore of bringing water from a well to his home using a bucket. However, the bucket had a hole in it. As the boy walked back to his house, unknowingly water would leak out through the hole. Despite his efforts, by the time he reached his home, the bucket would be nearly empty. Frustrated, the boy tried to walk faster, but no matter how quickly he moved, the water would still leak out. He tried carrying the bucket in different ways, but the result was always the same. Despite all his efforts, he could not prevent the water from leaking."

- The moral of the story is that instead of trying to work around a problem we need to address it at its root.

- In the case of the boy and his bucket, instead of finding ways to carry it faster, he needed only to plug the hole. This lesson reminds us that "slapping a bandaid" on a problem isn't enough. We often need to get past the symptoms and find the underlying cause of the problem. In the example of being "stuck in side control", it was really a guard retention problem. Instead of trying to leverage our strengths (carrying the bucket faster), we need to address our weaknesses (the hole in the bucket).

- True champions (on and off the mats), don't shy away from feedback, they seek it, understand it and embrace it.

- Feedback is the breakfast of champions because a true winner starts each day in search of personal growth. They nourish themselves with a steady diet of self-reflection and focused, corrective action. Just like a healthy diet fuels us for our day, feedback powers our journey towards self-mastery.

In BJJ your greatest teacher is your experiences on the mat. As you go further and deeper into this art you will begin to see the beautiful parallel's with your own life. The lessons on the mat, and how you face them, will echo the victories and failures in your own reality. **The way you handle that tough, unpredictable young purple belt can reflect on how you handle adversity in your day-to-day experiences.**

And just as the art of BJJ is often described as 'the gentle art,' the grace you display under pressure on the mats can inspire you to face life's challenges with the same poise and resilience, reminding us that true strength lies in our ability to remain composed and adaptable amidst the chaos.

Life in Entertainment:

One of my favorite "Seinfeld" episodes is called, "The Summer of George," where the concept of grace is discussed. In this episode Jerry Seinfeld's character is dating a professional ballerina. Throughout the episode, Jerry is enamored with her grace, poise, and elegance, qualities associated with her ballet profession. It is with great surprise that he discovers her "grace" doesn't extend beyond the dance floor.

In one scene, Jerry takes her out for dinner. She shockingly attacks the meal like a wild animal, which is in stark contrast to her elegant ballerina persona. He's shocked and remarks that he thought she would be "grace personified" in all aspects of her life.

The episode is a comedic commentary on the philosophy of "grace." It compels us to reevaluate how we perceive grace. It shows us that this quality is not inherent in all individuals across all situations. Rather it's a contextual, changeable quality that can be selectively applied. We all have access to grace. Have you heard the saying to "dig deep"? When you do, you may discover courage, but will likely find "grace."

Mission:

Look for opportunities to practice lessons while you're outside of the academy.

Take BJJ everywhere you go and let it shape your perspective and actions. Approach life with the mindset of finding creative solutions.

Recognize that everyone faces their own battles. Sharing BJJ isn't just about teaching the physical moves; it's about spreading its philosophy.

Note Taking

This is one of the most important skill sets for retention, and the least often used in Brazilian Jiu-Jitsu. Why is that? You might respond by saying, "Because I'm lazy?" No because you don't have a good system and haven't developed a habit around said system. It's really that simple. There's great power in regularly putting pen to paper. Just from a pragmatic stand point, it's almost impossible to remember everything you've been taught. There's too many moves and too much detail to keep it all. But note taking is a great way to record the important stuff and all the little details as well. You also begin to accumulate important data on your training and also reflect on your experiences.

Pen and Paper:

You have to first decide on your note taking method. If you're "old school" like me you might prefer writing it down. Writing notes engages the "encoding" process (transferring the information into a form that can be stored later) in your brain that allows you to store it at its deepest levels. The physical act of writing can help reinforce your memory retention. When you write something you engage fine motor skills. Experts agree that this physical act creates neural pathways in your brain. With writing you also have the benefit of adding drawings, diagrams, different colors, notes, etc.

Digital Note taking:

You can find Apps (applications) and software for note taking. They can be more versatile by offering the ability to access notes across all devices through cloud-based platforms.

Old School meets Digital:

"The Rocket book" works like a regular pen and notebook. It's a specially made notebook / journal that allows you to write on the pages and then scan a small QR code that places your notes into the cloud for later access. The pages can be easily erased as you go. I like this method as I get the best of both worlds. The pen writes really well and doesn't smudge. I personally recommend this system.

Apple iPhone Notes:

You can hand write your notes in a journal then take a picture of the notes. *The apple iPhone has an option that when you take a picture it will turn the words into useable text that you can 'copy' and 'paste' into your note pad. This is a great way to have the best of both worlds. You receive the value of writing it down with the benefit of having it stored digitally.

Take a picture of your notes:

With apple devices there's an option at the bottom right corner of the picture. It's a small icon of a four cornered outlined squares with three small lines in the center. Click on the icon and all of the words will be highlighted. Next select the text and then copy and paste it into a note.

Now that you have selected your note taking method, what do you write?

- First ask yourself, *what is the purpose of my notes?* They can be used as a personal archival record of your training experiences. You can write down descriptions of moves you're learning. Writing them out is like mental repetitions without physical movement. Experts say that your brain doesn't know the difference either. No matter how you slice it, reps are reps! If you're a beginner now, it will also be fun to look back on your notes when you're an upper belt in the future.

- You may choose to document each training session. Record the date you attended class, who taught and any specific techniques you learned. Break the techniques down into four simple steps.

For example:

Arm bar from guard -

1. Secure arm at the wrist and elbow

2. Place foot on hip / elevate and cut an angle

3. Leg covers head

4. Slide hands to the wrist and squeeze.

"**Chunking**," or breaking things into small manageable steps, has its origins in the field of cognitive psychology. It postulates that the brain can process information more efficiently when it is presented in smaller steps. The human brain has a limited volume to store and process information. According to studies, people have a working memory of between four and seven things. The "cognitive load", or the amount of mental work needed to absorb the information, is decreased when the task is broken into smaller pieces.

Through my experience of teaching kids and adults for many decades, I have seen this first hand. How do you teach a five year old an arm bar from the guard? The same way you teach a 40-year old. You do it in small, easy steps. But you cannot move onto the second step until you've mastered the first step, and so forth. If you follow this learning and teaching methodology you can "master" moves quicker. Why? Because you're no longer trying to absorb an entire move, but rather each individual step. The brain tends to perform better with four steps. Three isn't enough and five is too many. Four steps keeps it simple but with some room for details.

Assimilation happens through understanding. They are born of the same cloth.

- **Shuhari**, is a traditional Japanese martial arts teaching concept. It outlines the process of learning into three distinct stages.

- **Stage One "Shu"** - (White and blue belt) In this phase the students follows the steps of each technique without variation or question. There is a strict adherence to the "rules" of the move. This helps to build a solid groundwork of fundamental skills that are then built into muscle memory.

- **Stage Two "Ha"** - (purple and brown belt) At this level the student begins to experiment with new approaches and tailor the techniques to their body style, strengths, weaknesses and preferences. This is the stage of exploration, creativity and introspection.

- **Stage Three "Ri"** (black belt & beyond) When the student reaches the Ri level, they have progressed to the point of natural intuition. They have assimilated and embodied the core of the art and are free from the constraints of external rules and attachments. Because of this they can now influence the art itself.

The concept of Shuhari illustrates how crucial it is to learn the basics, experiment with different approaches, and then go beyond the norm in order to reach a level of actual mastery and genuine self-expression.

By utilizing this concept in your own BJJ you can begin to see how each stage of Shuhari is in direct correlation to truly understanding a technique. It seems to me that it is impossible to achieve mastery in all aspects of

Jiu-Jitsu. The art is infinite and the depth is too vast for complete assimilation. However, you may develop a high level of mastery in various aspects of Jiu-Jitsu. Your triangle game might be at a very high level of understanding, however your arm bar game might not be on par. Or maybe you're a white belt who just wants to survive and not be the nail forever. I can assure you, that won't be the case. Just keep telling yourself, "nobody sucks forever and everyone gets better."

- **One of the best hacks is taking good notes.** Do you want to get past the young buck at your BJJ gym? I can almost guarantee he doesn't take notes. That may seem like a small, fairly insignificant thing. It is not. You might not be able to beat him on the mats, however as a 40 plus practitioner, I bet you have far more discipline and maturity. This is your super power! Embrace it fully Ninja.

Note taking by skill level:

White belt note taking

As a beginner, your primary goal is to *learn and internalize* the techniques taught in class.

This includes positional hierarchy and terminology:

Guard, Side, Mount, Back. Secondary positions: half guard, north south, quarter guard, lock down, etc.

Example: *Day / Date / Instructor who taught*

Keep track of the warm-up drills and conditioning that you do in class -

This may inspire ideas for a home workout. Also record any new terminology that you may not have heard before. Look for oppor-tunities to connect the new moves you're learning to what you already know. This is called "**chaining**" in BJJ circles. It's a powerful learning modality because it allows you to expand on what you already know, while learning something new.

Goal setting -

As a beginner you can greatly benefit from setting both short-term and long-term goals for your BJJ development. Examples of goals: Next stripe on your belt, hit a specific technique rolling, tap someone who always taps you, roll more rounds, improve your flexibility, build more strength, improve cardio and endurance, etc.

Reflection -

Take some time to evaluate and reflect on your progress using your notes. Jot down your observations on each lesson, including any difficulties you had, any suggestions your teachers or training partners gave you, and any areas in which you feel you could use more work. This is the power of BJJ. When you do something wrong Jiu-Jitsu will tell you. There's an immediate feedback loop. You do it incorrectly and you pay the price for your mistake. (Bad position equals getting subbed, swept, taken down, etc.)

Review -

Establish a routine of reviewing your notes to really anchor the knowledge you're learning. You can also spend time updating and refreshing them regularly. You may want to add additional details to old techniques as you evolve your training. Using diagrams and sketches can aid in your note taking. Remember, if you can't draw well, don't feel bad. It's not an art contest!

Blue belt note taking

You have already mastered the basics of Brazilian Jiu-Jitsu and earned your blue belt in BJJ. The next step is to Quit! (No just kidding - the joke is every blue belt quits) The goal here is to hone your skills, experiment with new approaches and learn the fundamental principles and strategies behind your craft. If you want to get better at BJJ as a blue belt and prepare yourself for the next level, here are some tips for effective note taking.

Tip #1 - Seriously, Don't quit yet! (Blue belts are notorious for doing this)

As your BJJ game develops it will also become more complicated. You will want to organize your notes into specific technique categories. You can create sections for sweeps, counters, escapes, specific positions, sparring reflections, etc.

- Reflection - As a blue belt you will want to record the experience with each grappling partner. How did you do? What are you struggling with and where are your victories? Be specific.

- Keep track of all of your workouts - BJJ, weight training, endurance / cardio, etc. Monitor your personal progress and your partners. Where do they give you the most trouble? What are they good at, and how can you counter it? Focus on efficient breathing when you're rolling. Note how you physically feel after each round. Set both short-term and long-term goals and celebrate milestones.

Purple Belt note taking

"The me stage." Where a white belt is like a toddler, a purple belt is more like a teenager or even a young adult. You now have all the power of being a grown up, doing adult things, but you lack the life experience. This is important at this stage as you need to develop your "own" sense of identity with your own set of preferences. Much like a young adult aspiring to go to college, this is where you decide what you will be good at.

Purple belt is a great place to revisit and review old notes. This can help refresh old memories and inspire new ideas. Plus it will be fun to look back and appreciate the extent of your growth.

- Now that you've been training for a minute you can begin to play with other Jiu-Jitsu positions and attacks. You can build on your strengths while addressing your weaknesses. Make a list of every position or sequence that you feel weakest. Then develop solutions for each position. Ask the question, "How would I submit myself?" Then you can begin to fill in those gaps in your game.

- Broaden your own learning capacity. You can do this by trying new forms of skill acquisition. Go and try a seminar, visit an open mat in a nearby city, purchase an online course, set up a private lesson with a new coach or professor. Finding new ways of bringing BJJ into your life will give you greater insight.

- Analyze the game of high level competitors you admire. Find people who have a similar body style to yours. What techniques and strategies are working for them, and how can you make that applicable to your game?

- Building your mental game of Jiu-Jitsu. Take notes on how you feel during rolls. What is your emotional and mental state? If you're a competitor, ask yourself how do you feel during matches? Do you hit a state of flow? Or do you feel like you're drowning? Dive into these important, revealing questions.

Brown belt note taking

You're almost there now! Don't give up. Now is the time to become hyper focused on refining your game. You can no longer keep your blinders on about your BJJ. It's time to tear your game apart and build it back up. Explore your weaknesses and plug up all the "holes in your bucket."

- Self criticism will make you better. Begin to identify the gaps in your training while still appreciating your growth. Look for areas of expansion. If you are weak at leg attacks, then add them to your game. Wrist locks are your new toy at brown belt. Maybe it's now time to slap on some wrist locks and go full on prison rules.

- Brown belt is a great place to review and organize all of your old notes. If you're a paper and pen person, make sure you have them saved in a digital format as a back up.

- As an upper belt you may be given the opportunity to teach or assist in classes. Always have 2-3 class plans written and prepared for instances when you're called to fill in. If you haven't been asked, maybe it's because you haven't made your skills known. Let your professor know that you're available to help out if it's ever needed. Make notes on your teaching experiences and any feedback you've received. Continue to take notes on your mindset during classes, competitions and while teaching. Having a strong sense of self awareness will make you a better student and future professor.

- Network with others in the BJJ community both on and off-line. Support seminars at other dojos and seek out learning and teaching opportunities.

Black belt note taking

As a 40-plus BJJ black belt you have to make your health your life's mission. You cannot possibly help others if you're not in your best form. Use your BJJ notes for documenting all of your workouts. Record your weight training workouts, cardio, conditioning, stretching, etc. Having a place to document it will only reinforce the importance of doing it.

- You also want to focus on injury prevention and joint health more than ever. At your level you might have some wear on those tires. That's okay, make the appropriate adjustments. You can use your notebook to track your joints by writing down how you physically feel after each workout. For example: My elbow is hurting after I lift.

You can then look back and see where you may be contributing to something chronic.

- Pay close attention to how your body feels while practicing certain positions or techniques. You may notice knee pain while you're doing triangle chokes for example. In this case you start improving your hip flexibility and your knee pains may be resolved.

- Mental Exercise: As a BJJ black belt you have developed a vast library of techniques. Begin to isolate the four fundamental principles that bind every move together. This will simplify the teaching and learning process as you grow your pedagogy skills.

For example:

Armbar -

1. Isolate all three arm joints (wrist, elbow, shoulder)
2. Place your foot on the hip / raise your hips / cut an angle
3. Place your leg around the head
4. Chop your leg down as your raise your hips.

Of course your own steps to an arm bar might vary, but you get the point.

Add additional details to the move once you've isolated the four main steps. For example, how your body feels during the technique. Note any physical sensations. For example: "I felt my partner squeeze their legs around my arm thus causing the pressure from the trap to be amplified." Or on a triangle choke: "I notice that when I stomp my leg down and flair it away from my body I get a quicker tap." Once you have isolated the four steps to each move. Now try to **isolate the "secret sauce"** of each move. Just like the delicious sauce at "Chik-fil-a". No matter how nice you ask, nobody will tell you the recipe.

In my observation every move has a secret sauce. It's the one little thing (that becomes a big thing) that really advances the move and makes it nearly impossible to stop. For me, how you bite the neck with the back of your leg on the triangle that makes it the "secret sauce." Without the proper "bite", you are now forced to use strength in lieu of good technique.

Now that you're a BJJ black belt you have a vast amount of knowledge that is worth sharing. Schedule drilling time where you can dig into your notes and share techniques you're working on. Remember that the best way to assimilate something is to teach it to someone else. As a black belt teacher, document all of your class plans. This will give you an archival record of your classes for future reference and use.

As you progress in your training it is important to find a system of goal setting that works best for you. When it comes to setting goals there isn't a one size fits all method. It's really a personal thing.

Getting S.M.A.R.T

What I've found is that the SMART method is a simple blue print for goal attainment. It gained popularity in the 1980's and is still widely used today. For our purposes I have adapted it for an over 40 BJJ practice.

S.M.A.R.T. is an acronym for **Specific, Measurable, Attainable, Relevant, Time-bound**

S - Specific goals that answer three important questions. What? Why? How? What is your goal? Why do you want to achieve it? How will you accomplish it?

What - "I'm currently a two stripe white belt and I want to be a three stripe and eventually a blue belt."

Why - "If I were a blue belt I would feel more accomplished, in better health and be able to play the game of BJJ better."

How - "I will continue to train consistently three times per week. I will make sure I do whatever I can at home for good recovery. I will ensure I stay safe and injury free."

M - Measurable This asks the question of, "how will you track your goals and how will you know when you have reached them?"

"I will track my goals through consistent note taking. I will sit in my car and take notes before I leave after each class."

"I will seek the feedback from from training partners to gauge my growth and mat success."

"I will know that I have reached my goals because I will feel better physically and mentally and I will have my new belt tied proudly around my waist."

A - Attainable This asks the question, "Given your current constraints, is it possible to achieve your goals." Look at your life and determine if your current life, work, family schedule will lead you to your goals. Or do you need to make adjustments occasionally and recalibrate.

R - Relevant If you want to succeed, you need to set goals that matter to you personally. If something is important it will drive you to action in spite of obstacles. Ask yourself, "What techniques can I add to my BJJ game that will support and enhance what I am already doing?"

T - Time Bound Having a deadline around your goals will create urgency and focus. Left unattended your goals begin to collect dust and are soon forgotten. For example: "I want to earn my purple belt by XXX date." I am always concerned when someone says that they "don't care about the belts." I appreciate the sentiment. But in reality the belts in BJJ represent your personal evolution and point of progress. Belts aren't everything, but they do matter.

I was a brown belt for thirteen years. I know what it means to wait. I also know what it means to feel like you're not progressing. I'm often asked, "What caused your eventual breakthrough?" It was when I hyper focused on achieving my BJJ black belt and doing all of the things that it required. That meant getting myself in the best physical condition, earning my professors respect by successfully competing, and learning all of that curriculum that was required of me.

Don't discount the value of the belts as it can be a useful tool for growth. Just remember, it's always about the journey and not the destination. Or as Mr. Miyagi said, "In Okinawa, belt mean no need rope to hold up pants."

Mission:

Good note taking is really about having a good system and habit. Once you decide 'how' you'll take notes, you will then need to decide when and where you'll exercise this powerful new habit. In your car before you leave your academy is a great place to start. This way the content from class is still fresh in your mind. The more time that passes, the fewer details will be remembered.

Psychologist Hermann Ebbinghaus's research on the 'forgetting curve' suggests that memory of new material rapidly declines over the 24 hours following exposure to it. The key point, however, is that this decline can be mitigated if the material is reviewed in some fashion. When you **write down your class notes while they're fresh you're less likely to forget the important stuff**. As you know in BJJ everything is important. Your notes should also reflect where you are in your training. If you're are blue belt, then utilize the suggestions for note taking at your level.

You'll also want to schedule some review Pomodoro's. Set a reminder in your phone for a twenty minute review session of your notes. You can use this time to quiz yourself on your new moves. You can review the four steps to the technique, then without looking, speak them aloud. (If you're in a public place, maybe say them in your head) Your notes are also a great place to set and review your goals. The SMART method is a simple guideline to goal setting. Your goals can be related to both BJJ and your personal life. As you advance in your Jiu-Jitsu training, you'll start to notice significant similarities between BJJ and your everyday life. It's important not to overlook the relevance of these parallels.

Finding Your Learning Style

If you want to become an efficient and effective student it helps to identify your preferred learning styles. Below you will find the various learning types. In addition, you can adopt other learning styles as well. **V.A.R.K.** is an acronym for Visual, Auditory, Reading / Writing, Kinesthetic learners.

Visual - They need to see things done visually. Mind maps (flow charts), colored pens, drawings and illustrations, all can help with retention.

Auditory - They benefit from verbal explanations, audio books, and pneumonic devices based on sound and rhythm.

Reading / Writing - They benefit using written language to learn.

Kinesthetic - They are the classic hands on learner.

It's vital to remember that *most people don't only rely on one learning style* but use a variety of them. Understanding how to utilize your preferred learning style can fuel your success. Let's get into some specific tips on how to use your learning style to advance your progress.

Visual Learners -

You will find that you learn best by seeing someone demonstrate a technique. Viewing instructional videos and online course can be an excellent option. You may find it helpful to turn down the volume as you watch the video. I am a visual learner myself so I tend to watch videos with no audio.

BJJ practitioners can also benefit from the visual organization and analysis provided by flow charts. A flow chart provides a visual representation of how moves connect together.

You can create a flow chart using one large piece of paper or a smaller sheet. Start with a small box in the center and record your first move.

For example:

Choose your starting point -

Locked closed guard

(Next draw an arrow to your next move) ——->

Hip bump sweep——> Mount——> Cross Collar Choke ——->

Partner does Upa —> Back to guard, finish with cross collar choke

The point is to connect one box to the next to create a continuous stream of attacks and counters. You can add additional branches to each box to create alternative steps and counters. This will take your flow chart in multiple directions with differentiating sequences.

You can make your flow chart more readable and understandable by color-coding or using symbols to denote the various types of attacks (such as submissions, escapes, sweeps and counters). Regularly review and update your flow chart. This is a stellar exercise regardless of your learning style.

Auditory Learners -

In this modality you learn best from verbal presentations. Where the visual learner turns the volume down, the auditory learner wants to hear every important detail. When you watch videos try viewing them wearing ear phones to eliminate distractions. You may find it effective to close your eyes and listen without viewing from time to time. When you physically practice a move it will be helpful to audibly speak the steps as you do them. As you do this remember key aspects of each move and say them aloud.

For example:

On a triangle choke you might cue yourself by saying,

"Hand on head, postures down, stomp and squeeze."

These verbal cues will help you anchor the steps and create muscle memory.

- Make use of pneumonic devices to help you remember the important details. For example when you take the back: "Harness before hooks." This will help you to remember to secure a seatbelt before you attempt your hooks.

A few good BJJ pneumonic devices:

- **"Harness before hooks"** - For when you have someone's back and you want to establish upper body control before putting getting your hooks (legs) around their body.

- **"You need a seat belt grip to take a trip"** - This references the concept of getting control of your partners back from the turtle position. Without a seatbelt you will lose control.

- **"A.B.C. Always Be Choking"** - This refers to the concept of always looking for and attacking your opponents neck.

- **"B.A.S.E."** Balance Alignment Structure Efficiency" (when referring to maintaining positional control) - You must keep your body securely in-balance so not to be swept or reversed. In side control your alignment would be how you position your body in reference to your partners. Generally from side control you're perpendicular to your partner (not parallel)

- The Alphabet Game - Assign a move to each letter of the alphabet to see how many you know. A -Armbar, B - Baseball choke, Cross collar choke, D - Darce choke, etc.

Alliteration is the repetition of the same consonant sounds at the beginning of words in a sentence. For example: "Grab, Grip, Go" They all begin with the letter "G" which creates rhythm when you speak it. For auditory learners this is especially helpful. The repeated sound makes it more memorable and easier to call upon when needed.

Here's some examples of alliterative phrases:

Guard Passes

Grip, Grab, Go for a sweep - Relating to setting up a guard sweep.

Posture, Pressure, Pass the guard - A reminder to have good posture and pressure to pass the guard.

Base, Balance, Break the guard - relative to making sure that your legs are under you for good base when you're passing the guard.

Sweeps

Butterfly breaks the base and boosts - On a butterfly sweep you want to disrupt their base and to lift and load them for the sweep.

Hips high, hook and heave - On a hip bump sweep you want to elevate your hips, hook their arm and sweep them.

Lift for leverage and launch - This is a great reminder that you have to load your partners body weight in order to sweep them.

Submissions

Triangle traps, tightens and taps - Referring to a triangle choke. You must keep your lock tight and never release pressure until you get the tap.

Armbar angle, hips high, chop and apply - On a guard armbar you want to create an angle, elevate your hips to their arm, chop down with the leg covering the head and then apply leverage.

Control, constrict, choke - On the rear naked choke its important to maintain control of the neck, and slowly constrict the blood flow to get a proper strangle.

Now have some fun creating some of your own phrases that relate to your BJJ game.

Reading and Writing learning style

With this learning modality you retain information quicker through linguistics and writing exercises. Making use of note taking, drawings and diagrams can be helpful. I have had great success with teaching students to use BJJ flash cards. Draw or write the name of a technique on one side. On the other side write out a description of the move or the four steps necessary to execute it. You can then quiz yourself on various moves. Try this immediately after class, later that same day, same week and month and so on.

- Journaling about your Jiu-Jitsu can help you to reflect and grow as a practitioner. You can write out descriptions of matches you've had, especially if you're a competitor. You can even do this before a competition to help you set the tone for your experience.

- Another great method of learning moves is to teach them to others. Teaching allows you to learn to articulate the moves so others can understand them on a deeper level. This will expand your own ability to absorb them as well. Teaching is drilling!

As a reading and writing learner, you will find BJJ books beneficial. Both reading and listening to books, podcasts or videos will entertain and inspire you.

Kinesthetic Learners

I personally happen to be a combination of a visual and kinesthetic learner. I find that when I watch the moves first and then immediately execute it, I retain the moves quicker. The ability to get your hands dirty and have a tactile experience is imperative for kinesthetic people.

- Drill, drill and drill some more. For the hands on person you need to get your physical reps in to build muscle memory. The more you practice, the quicker your body will internalize them. **Try doing reps with your eyes close**d. Removing the external distractions and stimulation will expand your internal focus. When one sense is removed the others become more profound.

- Collaborate closely with your training partners and solicit their input on how to improve your reps. Don't get sloppy. If your repetitions start to degrade in technique, your partner needs to let you know. **Poor practice is often far worse than no practice**. You don't want to reinforce bad habits. Know how to work hard, but also when to stop.

- Another great option is to **consider private lessons if it fits into your budget**. You pay more for one-on-one instruction, but it's usually worth it. You're getting your professor or another high ranking students immediate feedback. Not only do they see your technique first hand, they feel it. That alone is invaluable.

- Volunteer as an UKE (receiver of the move) whenever possible. Being able to feel your teachers technique, pressure, weight distribution, etc. is extremely helpful. Always be the first to raise your hand with questions and with offering yourself as a volunteer. Being an UKE is both an honor and opportunity. If you want to be chosen by your teacher, let them know. But also make sure you can fulfill the role appropriately. You want to keep your body relaxed but fully engaged. The TORI (giver of the move) can't properly demonstrate a move if you're a limp noodle. Conversely they too cannot perform the move if you're a brick house either. Try to receive the move without overly anticipating it or completely fighting it. There's a balance that happens between the TORI and the UKE. It's a dance not to be taken lightly.

Mission:

Start by identifying how you learn best. What combination of learning styles do you prefer? Would you be willing to expand your learning styles? By understanding your preferred style you will enhance and speed up the process of automaticity. By increasing your learning styles, you can create a more fluid Jiu-Jitsu experience. In some cases your professor may teach in a way that only addresses one or two learning styles. This can be frustrating when you're a beginner (or anyone) trying to learn something new. By understanding and expanding how you learn, you can adapt to different teaching methods and enhance your ability to grasp Jiu-Jitsu techniques more effectively. **By diversifying your own learning styles you become open to all teaching modalities**. You can explore this by trying a new learning style.

For example:

If you are not an auditory learner, try not looking at the screen and only listen to the technique. Over time you can improve your listening skills. Play with this expansion concept!

- Try utilizing alliterative phrases for remembering Jiu-Jitsu techniques, key points and strategies. You can use the options we've supplied or create some of your own relating to your BJJ game. This is also a great way to remember new steps or sequences. You can document these in your BJJ notebook.

- Finally for this mission, volunteer to be an "UKE" (receiver of the move) in class. This will help you feel exactly what your professor is doing when performing a technique. If you are a lower belt and there's not an option to be the UKE. You can have your professor do the move on you when they're making the rounds for corrections. Simply ask, "Would you mind doing it on me so I can feel it?" But be prepared for what you're inviting. They may give it a little extra squeeze so you can "feel it."

Improving Your Memory

Your mind is a powerful tool, when used correctly it can accelerate your BJJ learning ability. When it comes to consolidating and remembering new material, the human brain is unparalleled. According to experts, our minds can potentially hold as much data as 2.5 petabytes (1024 terabytes or a million gigabytes). That's the same as keeping a TV recording going for around 300 years straight. If you're like me you're saying, "Nope I can't remember what I ate for lunch, so I definitely can't do complicated BJJ moves!" Don't worry, you're not alone. Just like every other part of our body, our brain ages as we age. The good news is, it isn't all bad news. There's a lot we can do to improve our brain health.

Here's a list of foods and supplements that can improve brain health:

Green tea - Caffeine and rich in antioxidants. Matcha green tea is also excellent for brain health. Research has shown that compounds in matcha can enhance brain function.

Blueberries - High in antioxidants.

Dark chocolate - contains caffeine, flavonoids and antioxidants.

Turmeric - Curcumin, the main ingredient, has anti-inflammatory and antioxidant properties and has been demonstrated to pass the blood-brain barrier, suggesting it may enhance memory and mood.

Pumpkin seeds - Contains micro nutrients that can improve brain function.

Omega 3's (fish oil) - Antioxidant and anti-inflammatory effects.

Nootropics - They are substances that promise to boost cognitive processes like memory, creativity, focus, and motivation. They can be found as a dietary supplement.

Caffeine - Improves mood and increase energy. Some studies have shown that it can improve reaction time, problem solving and memory consolidation.

Mushrooms - Not the magic ones, but these can have magical results.

Lions Mane - Studies show it can stimulate growth of brain cells.

Chaga - Anti-inflammatory effects, supports immune health.

Reishi - Immune support and neuroprotective effects.

Cordyceps - Some studies suggest that they may have anti-aging effects and can improve memory function.

Like most things in life, consistency is the key that unlocks potential. The quickest path to mastery is through repetition. Do something enough times and it becomes second nature. Think of riding a bike or driving a car. You don't think about every muscle, movement, etc. that is involved. You just ride a bike. The term "muscle memory" is commonly used to refer to our muscles' innate capacity to recall and automatically reproduce previously performed actions. However, keep in mind that **it is the brain, and not the muscles that store the information.**

When we acquire a new skill, like an armbar, the brain creates new connections that coordinate the newly acquired skill. Initially when you learn something new it requires conscious effort to perform the sequences correctly. This is why we break moves down into small, digestible chunks. It's far easier to learn a few small steps than to master an entire sequence of moves.

Through conscious, repetitive practice, the brain builds neural connections. This is known as "neuroplasticity", the brains ability to reorganize and alter its structure in response to new experiences. Quite literally to stretch the possibilities.

As we continue to drill and have experiences around the new move, the need to consciously think about it becomes greatly reduced and eventually streamlined. It's like catching a ball. If someone threw a ball at you, you would instinctively try to catch it. You wouldn't examine the angle, speed and force of the throw. You would extend your hand and attempt to catch it. Through time and practice the communication (time gap) between the brain and the muscles becomes instantaneous. You've probably heard of the 10,000 rule. It purposes that an athlete must perform around 10,0000 deliberate repetitions of something in order to develop mastery.

The key isn't "10,000" but rather, "deliberate."

The definition of deliberate is "something being done consciously and intentionally." You can't just bang out twenty armbars and expect to now "get it" under hostile conditions. But on the other side, who has the time to do a move for 10,000 reps. Neither is realistic. So the question then is, "How does someone practice BJJ and learn all of these complicated moves without spending a lifetime doing it?" Yes you need to do a lot of reps, but it's not *JUST* a numbers game. You have to go deeper down the rabbit hole. **It's not 'how many you do', but how you are doing them that matters most.**

Can you DTP?

How do you know that you've got a move down and can move onto something new? I follow three criteria for every move. I call it the **DTP formula. Demonstrate. Teach. Perform**

Can you demonstrate it? Can you teach it? Have you performed it successfully live?

- Question one asks can you demonstrate the move? This demands whether you can execute the technique, smoothly and without hesitation, for someone else. If they had never seen the move before could you demonstrate it in a way that they could understand it by watching it without any spoken instructions? This is vital because if you cannot, then you can't move onto step #2.

- For question number two you have to be able to successfully teach it to someone else. Now that you can demonstrate the move, can you translate it in a way that someone whose never seen it before can learn it? That means that you can break the move down into smaller pieces that someone can acquire, regardless of their skill level. Remember, that the more that you teach something, the better you get at it. Teaching is like learning on steroids.

- Once you're confident in teaching it to others you need to pressure test it over and over. This will help you work out any kinks while under hostile conditions. It allows you to become intimate with the move and make appropriate adjustments and tweaks. You now know it inside and out.

Building mental fortitude in BJJ isn't just about toughing it out; it's about cultivating a mindset that embraces learning, resilience, and adaptability. Techniques to boost your mental game include:

Practicing being fully present during each roll. Focus on your breathing, movements, and reactions to stay grounded and calm under pressure. Regularly visualize successful execution of techniques and winning scenarios to build confidence and reinforce neural pathways. Train your brain to see mistakes as learning opportunities. Adapt your strategies based on what the mat teaches you each day.

Emotional Regulation: Keep your emotions in check—don't let frustration or ego dictate your rolls. Use setbacks as fuel to drive your commitment to improve.

Mission:

Incorporate brain-boosting foods and supplements into your diet—like green tea, blueberries, and omega-3s. Prioritize consistent, deliberate practice of your BJJ techniques using the DTP formula: Demonstrate, Teach, Perform. This method not only ingrains the movements into your muscle memory but also strengthens your cognitive abilities through active learning and adaptation. Make each practice session count by focusing on the quality of your repetitions and seeking to understand the mechanics behind each move deeply.

Survival Expert: CLARK GREGG

BJJ Black Belt awarded by Renato Magno in 2015

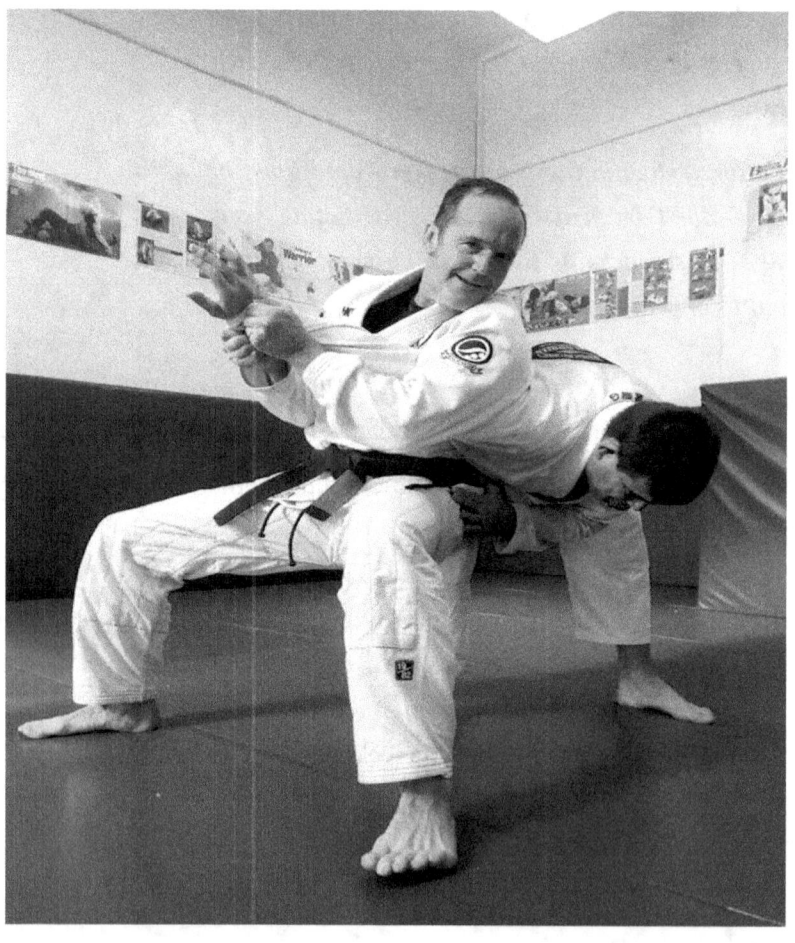

Intel:

He is an American actor, screen writer and director. He is well known for playing Phil Coulson on TV and in films for the Marvel Cinematic Universe. He has starred in numerous films and TV shows with a long career in the entertainment industry. He has also showcased his skills behind the camera with his incredible versatility in directing and screenwriting.

From the Source:

When you turn 40 you notice changes in your strength, your flexibility, your endurance. True in your body, true in your life. Some people take that as a sign to slow down. But that only accelerates the process.

I hate to work out, but I love to play.

I love to learn and improve.

I found Jiu-Jitsu at 40 and as anyone whoever has trained will tell you, there's always more to learn and room to improve. There are plenty of sessions that are incredibly humbling, but there are others where you get lost in the flow, the transitions, and you find that time has stopped. Or at least slowed down a little.

In Jiu-Jitsu, every instinct you have wants to do everything but relax or breathe when someone's attacking you, and learning that takes a long time. I think that's why a lot of people stop at blue belt because it's really hard to do. It's hard to take that next step. It took me a long time.

Imposter Syndrome

Impostor syndrome is a pattern in a person's mind in which they question their skills, talents, or accomplishments and have a constant fear of being found out as a "fraud." Even though others can clearly see their excellence. Those who experience this phenomenon still think they are fakes and don't deserve the success that they have achieved.

"I have written eleven books, but each time I think, 'uh oh, they're going to find out now. I've run a game on everybody, and they're going to find me out.'" -Maya Angelou

Towards the end of his life Albert Einstein once remarked, *"the exaggerated esteem in which my lifework is held makes me very ill at ease. I feel compelled to think of myself as an involuntary swindler."*

I have heard many BJJ students over the years express this same sentiment. "I don't deserve to be a blue belt... or purple belt...or... You fill in the blank." It's more common than you think that your fellow teammates think they aren't that good at BJJ. You may then be saying, "Well if they think they suck and they're tapping me. What does that say about me?"

The answer is, nothing. The truth is everyone sucks at BJJ at first (or for a while). But there is a breaking off point where some are just better than others. You first start to see these discrepancies at blue belt. Some people just pick things up quicker than others. But ultimately the technology of Jiu-Jitsu prevails and everyone has a breakthrough. In fact, this will undoubtedly happen multiple times in your journey.

But why do some people feel like they're a failure when they are actually experiencing success (even if it's slowly)? Imposter syndrome is believed to have its roots in early childhood experiences. If you were raised by parents who were perfectionists and had high expectations, this may be a contributing factor.

As an adult it can rear its head in your own BJJ experience. When students say, "I don't care about belts and stripes." I see it as a red flag. I understand the sentiment that the training is the most important thing. Not the "reward" of the belt or a physical piece of tape. It's important to acknowledge that stripes and belts do matter. Like it or not, they are the stick by which we measure our progress.

The belts aren't the perfect metric, but they do work. I can tell a healthy colored belt program at a BJJ academy when everyone is fairly close in skill level. In other words, there aren't huge discrepancies in competence. You'll always have a few people who are naturally gifted and a few who are not. There should be an average ability level at each belt. When we talk about imposter syndrome this is where we see it most. Students who feel like they don't deserve their belt, or who miss promotions and tests on purpose under the guise that belts don't matter.

I have also observed students with imposter syndrome experience challenges with performance anxiety. This can play itself out in executing techniques at formal tests and while competing in tournaments. Even when they perform well they will attribute it to luck or happenstance. If you've had this experience, remind yourself of the small victories you have made along the way. Remember, every success doesn't have to be a medal, trophy or belt. It can be the small experiences on the mat that we share with our training partners.

Examples of 'Small Celebrations':

"The fact that I am over 40 and training BJJ is awesome!"

"I am over 40 and completing. Win or lose, I am doing it!"

"Whatever rank you are right now is better than before you started when you were a No Belt"

"I don't have to tap everyone, every time. But each time I show up I am tapping everyone who chose to stay home"

"My age is my asset"

"My courage to step on the mats is a testament to my strength"

"I am patient and progress takes time"

"I welcome feedback as a tool for growth"

"Every day I show up, I am one step closer to my goals"

"I learn from every roll"

"I am building resilience with every roll"

"Even when it's not fun, it's still fun"

"My age is my superpower"

"It's a small piece of tape, but a huge leap in confidence"

"I bring wisdom to the mats"

Spend some time creating affirmations that focus on the 'small wins' that lead to the big victories. Create a list of BJJ related goals and attach affirmations to each objective.

Goal: I want to be a BJJ black belt.

Affirmation: **"I move with the ease and efficiency of a black belt"**

Goal: I want to successfully compete in a BJJ tournament.

Affirmation: **"It feels so good to confidently compete!"**

Goal: To not feel anxiety around going to BJJ class.

Affirmation: **"I am allowed to be a beginner and make mistakes"**

Goal: To feel confident about going to BJJ class.

Affirmation: **"My BJJ progress is measured in persistence not perfection"**

Goal: To earn my next BJJ belt or stripe.

Affirmation: **"Every class I attend is one step closer to my goal"**

Goal: To keep going.

Affirmation: **"I show up and try every time and that is enough"**

Goal: To stay injury free.

Affirmation: **"My body speaks and I listen"**

Goal: To release anxiety about class.

Affirmation: **"The butterflies I feel are my bodies way of showing excitement!"**

Goal: To not quit.

Affirmation: **"Even on the tough days I'm still growing and learning"**

Goal: To win your first competition medal.

Affirmation: **"I am ready and deserving of success"**

By embracing a growth mindset you begin to realize that failure is part of the journey. It helps you eliminate all the bad habits that don't serve you. When you celebrate your strengths and face your weaknesses you have no choice but to become better. It's okay to have growing pains, but we don't need to suffer through them.

Mission:

Track progress by consistent effort, resilience, and the willingness to learn from every experience.

Balancing Principle and Conceptual Based Learning

Another great force for assimilating moves is applying a conceptual approach to learning BJJ. By following a more abstract way of thinking you can begin to understand techniques from a broader context. With a Principle based learning approach you will focus on the underlying details that govern BJJ.

"If you give a man a fish, you feed him for a day. If you teach a man to fish, you feed him for a lifetime." In BJJ terms, "**If you teach someone an armbar from one position, they have one technique for one scenario. Teach them the broader concept, and they have a lifetime of techniques.**"

What is the broader concept of an armbar? In short, It's that the arm has three joints (wrist, elbow and shoulder). When leverage is applied from a fulcrum, you can dislocate the joint. If it can be done from all four positions. So instead of thinking of it as an armbar from the mount. Think of it as a joint manipulation.

Let's imagine you are putting a puzzle together, but without a picture to work from. You just have a blank box full of puzzle pieces. You have no visual reference. You would probably start with the outside pieces and create a frame and then fill in the middle portion. Little by little a picture would form from the connected puzzle pieces.

Conceptual BJJ is very similar. You work from a bigger framework which allows you to be more adaptable in the present moment. As great as muscle memory is, there are potential drawbacks.

I'll share a story to illustrate this point. I'm not sure if its leftovers from my mid 90's hacky sack days but I like to catch things with my feet. It's why I enjoy working from the guard. I love the idea of using my feet like hands. It makes me feel like a monkey. I've even do drills from time-to-time where I catch balls with my feet from varying distances. This "skill" developed into me instinctively catching things on the top of my feet. You know you drop your toothbrush and catch it on the top of your foot when it's falling. That sort of thing. A few years ago I was filling up my water bottle at a water tank. You know the ones you see in an office environment with the huge five gallon water bottle resting on top. As I was filling it I fell forward and knocked off the water container on top. As it tumbled to the floor below, I instinctively stuck out my foot to catch it! I think you know how the story ends. My fragile metatarsal bones could not withstand the weight of almost five gallons of water. Yep, I broke my foot. This is muscle memory gone array. I had integrated this response of catching things on my feet so strongly that I couldn't consciously adapt when I needed to.

When you rely too heavily on pre-programmed moves, you literally cannot get out of your own way. **Adaptation requires conscious thinking**. When you are constantly running a series of patterns, they become habitual. As we know, a good habit is hard to break. We want to strike a balance between principle / detail based learning and conceptual techniques.

The truth is we need a little bit of both. The advantage with muscle memory is that we don't have to think about every little step to execute the move correctly. We can move our thoughts onto other more important areas. The perfect balance would be to use your muscle memory to execute the move but stay consciously alert to the ever-changing environment. Always be hyper aware of moments for adaptability.

You can merge both worlds through various drilling techniques:

Drill #1 -

"Switch drill" - Start in your partners closed guard and begin your normal passing routines as your partner gives you varying levels of resistance and road blocks. Keep flowing though positions etc. but when your partner says "switch" you have to change gears and do something different. Preferably something you don't normally do. This will allow for creativity and adaptability on the fly.

Drill #2 -

"Bad day at the office" - Start from non-dominant positions. For example you might have your partner start from your back with both hooks and a harness. The goal is to add progressive resistance from the attacker. This allows for creativity and problem solving in compromising positions without getting injured.

Drill #3 -

"Really bad day at the office" - With this drill you have to err on the side of caution and be very mindful with your pressure and leverage. Start from a submission and practice your escape strategies while being open to new opportunities. *Never lock out submissions and go at around 20 - 30% effort. This keeps everyone safe while allowing for creative exploration.

Drill #4 -

"Flow Chain" When you chain moves together in BJJ you create a series of interconnected movements. This is important because it creates depth and confusion for your partner. If you attack with one thing, they can easily defend it. But when it becomes a series of moves built around predictable responses, it becomes insurmountable.

With this drill you will flow roll with your partner. Be sure to maintain structure in your body (don't be a noodle) but also don't offer complete resistance either. Find that balance of opposition and cooperation. As you flow with your partner, your goal is to locate your favorite submissions, sweeps and escapes. This gives you a chance to move freely in an unpredictable fashion, while finding familiarity along the way. Even try to hit your favorite moves from places and positions you wouldn't normally find yourself.

By combining concept based learning into muscle memory you broaden your understanding and application of new skills.

Mission:

Blend detailed, principle-based drilling with broader conceptual understanding. Merge conceptual foundations with muscle memory and refine your execution as well as stay alert and adaptable to the dynamic nature of live sparring. This model encourages you to think on your feet and apply principles creatively across various scenarios, improving your overall grappling intelligence and effectiveness on the mats.

Dunning-Kruger and Cognitive Load

The Dunning-Kruger effect is a cognitive bias where individuals with little or no ability about a subject vastly overestimate their ability or knowledge about it. It's like when someone says they know a lot about something, but really know nothing. You might say it's the opposite of imposter syndrome.

The story behind this phenomena is one of the craziest I have ever heard. As the story goes, McArthur Wheeler was a Pittsburgh man who believed he could rob a bank undetected by putting lemon juice on his face in lieu of a mask. His belief was based on the idea that lemon juice could be used as an invisible ink. He thought he could apply it to his face and not be seen by security cameras. In 1995, he robbed two banks in Pittsburgh during the day, without a mask or any other cover. He did this because he was sure that the lemon juice would hide his face from the cameras. Surveillance video made it easy to figure out who he was, and he was arrested the very same day. When Wheeler saw the video, he was shocked and allegedly said, "But I wore the juice."

This story caught the attention of social psychologists David Dunning and Justin Kruger. They viewed Wheeler as the perfect example of someone who is both bad at their job but not competent enough to realize it. This became the impetus of their research. Just like we see imposter syndrome playing out in BJJ, the Dunning-Kruger effect has also found it's home on the mats. But what causes us to think in this way? Experts believe it is caused by poor self-awareness or low metacognition. You can think of metacognition as the ability to judge one's own performance at a task. Because they don't know what they don't know, they tend to over-estimate their knowledge.

Metacognition is often described as "thinking about thinking" and can be broken down into two key areas:

Metacognition knowledge -

The ability to understand how you learn best. For example if you are a visual, auditory, reading / writing or kinesthetic learner? It also relates to understanding how you learn most effectively.

Metacognitive skills -

This refers to the strategies an individual uses to perform a task. This includes monitoring your own personal understanding and comprehension of whether a strategy is working.

The first, metacognition knowledge can be further broken down into the following:

personal knowledge, task knowledge and strategy knowledge. Think of personal knowledge as the conversation going on in your head while you roll. Task knowledge is the physical act of grappling or performing a technique. Whereas strategy knowledge is the game plan you're trying to adhere to while rolling or executing a move.

Beginner's often experience the Dunning-Kruger effect by over-estimating their skill level and underestimating what it takes to advance in Jiu-Jitsu. This can appear as the "spazzy white belt" who goes too fast, ends up getting hurt and quits. In other cases, it can slow the learning process dramatically. It can also appear when students under estimate what it takes to progress (whether in belts or learning techniques). Often times beginners expect to get immediate, positive feedback. But as we know, the opposite is true. The mats will only reflect exactly where you are today. "Fake it to make it" does not work in Jiu-Jitsu. The mats do not lie, nor should you. To get better at anything, especially a complicated martial art like Brazilian Jiu-Jitsu, you have to practice often, be patient, and know that the journey is just as important as the destination. Remember, a tree starts out as a small seed. You cannot rush the process, but you can slow it down. By the way, slowing things down is often the quickest way to assimilate moves (or building lasting muscle memory). Newer students tend to want to drill a technique too fast too soon. Speed is usually the final part of the equation. When you attempt to drill new moves fast they get sloppy, incoherent and are often executed wrong. Drilling fast requires muscle memory which doesn't happen at the beginning stages of a technique.

In the chapter on note taking we broke down the Japanese concept of "**Shuhari**." The first phase, "Shu" means to obey or adhere to the rules of the technique. This is the beginning stage of learning where the core concepts are driven home. Think of an armbar, for example, it has four fundamental steps.

1. Secure the arm,
2. Place your foot on the hip
3. Create an angle and chop your leg down on the back of the neck
4. Elevate your hips while squeezing your thighs together.

The goal is to master each step and to only advance forward when the previous step is done correctly and with complete control. Let's say you started the armbar and had the arm secured, but as you created your angle you lost a good portion of the arm. Can you advance to step number three? No.

If you tried to continue to step three, you would most likely lose the move and position. This is precisely what happens to inexperienced grapplers. They either don't have the steps memorized or mastered and try to do the move but they fail. This is why I break every move down into four steps. Once the first four steps are absorbed, then we add more details but always in the format of "four steps." The brain will better absorb the techniques when they're presented in simple, digestible chunks.

This is supported by the "**cognitive load theory**" of learning. It is based on the idea that our working memory, where we handle information, has a limited amount of space. The theory describes three types of cognitive load:

Intrinsic load - Think of this as where you are starting from. Do you have any previous knowledge of the task at hand? Are you familiar with what you're learning? This will be affected by the learners skill level. An armbar from the mount has a lower intrinsic load for a purple belt than a new white belt.

- What can you do? Start by identifying and memorizing the four steps assigned to every BJJ move. By breaking things down into smaller incremental steps you can maximize your learning. Remember, you cannot advance forward with a step until the previous steps have been performed with complete control and understanding.

- What can an instructor do? Present material in simple, easy to understand steps. Don't overcomplicate techniques and know your audience. Do they have any previous experience with this technique? Instructors can utilize an 'incremental learning' strategy where moves build on one another.

Extraneous load - This is created by how the information is presented. If the teacher doesn't follow a plan and jumps all the over the place this can further slow down the learning process. Think of this as all the "extra, non-essential, BS" that can come from a poorly executed class plan. This seems to be fairly common in BJJ classes. Inexperienced instructors often teach from the cuff. Just going with what they're feeling or excited about that day. I used to be just this way, until I realized that my students would progress more fluidly with an organized plan.

- What can you do? Mindful learning can be effective. Focus completely on what the instructor is presenting and avoid internal and external distractions. Clarify any points not understood by the instructor before advancing forward with the technique.

- What can an instructor do? Plan your classes and build on previous material. Demonstrate moves from various angles and use simple, easily understood language. Impress your students with your straight forward explanations, don't over complicate anything. Teach it so a five year old can understand it!

Our third load phase is called "**Germane load**" (In Latin Germanus, meaning genuine). This refers to the memory involved in the process of learning itself. This is the 'how' of learning. Think of it as the strategies and systems that are employed to acquire the new skill. You can also think of germane as being derived from the word "germinate." In the botanical context, germinate refers to the sprouting of stems, leaves and roots. This has a powerful metaphorical meaning as it suggests the birth of an idea, plan or system from its beginning stages. I often ask my own students at the conclusion of a class, "what will you do with he seed you have been given?" The line of thought I am trying to provoke is, what will you now do with the new move you have been given?

- What can you do? This can be note taking, videoing the moves in class (either when your professor is demonstrating them, or yourself performing them on a training partner), or any other strategy that helps you acquire the moves. Don't passively learn, ask questions as they arise. Keep detailed notes for later. Schedule a time for reflection and mental rehearsal (visualization). At the very minimum, write out your four steps to the technique. The first 24 hours is the key as the further you get from the source material, the harder it will be too mentally recover. By acting right away, you're encoding the material. Remember, encoding is the process by which the material can be stored for later retrieval. With fresh, new content time is of the essence.

- What can an instructor do? By linking new techniques to older techniques you can maximize a student's learning potential. Encourage students to ask questions and seek feedback from one another. If you're comfortable, allow them to video moves as they're presented. This gives them them the perfect archival reference for later retrieval. You can also allow students to video each other, to provide real-time feedback.

The aim of cognitive load theory in the context of BJJ is to manage all three load phases. The goal as an instructor is to minimize and eliminate the extraneous load by simplifying the presentation of techniques. By using clear, concise language and breaking moves into four steps, you can also better manage the intrinsic load. Of the three, the germane phase may be the most crucial. This is because it leads you to deep learning, which is the ultimate goal of assimilation.

You can think of deep learning as the "knowing" of a technique versus pure memorization. This includes the retention and performance of moves under hostile and ever-changing environments. This is important in BJJ as grappling matches are often referred to as "physical chess." Just like its counterpart, BJJ requires an effective strategy, problem solving, adaptability on the fly, and creative innovation. These can only be reached through deep learning.

Nothing can replace regular practice to improve muscle memory. Just like we discussed the importance of minimizing our extraneous load, we need to do that on a physical level as well. It's important to maximize learning potential by eliminating everything that creates barriers to it. Just like the farmer who prepares his land before seeding it. You too must create the best conditions to facilitate growth.

Often times the roadblocks we face are mostly self-imposed. We may look around and see others learning moves faster and having better results and wonder, is it me? It's probably a little bit of both. We can't deny our partner their own physical and mental attributes and personal progression. Yes they may sometimes be faster, younger or stronger. But aside from those attributes mentioned, why do others appear to learn things quicker?

It may seem "faster" but often it's our own barriers to learning that are slowing the process. We may just be doing a poor job preparing our fields for harvest. In this section I will share examples of where we may be failing ourselves and what can be done about it.

Consistency in the key that unlocks potential. I have preached this concept to my own students for as long as I can remember. (I'll probably mention it a few times in this book) The truth is that potential is nothing absent of action. A rock has potential. It can be used to create or destroy. Or it can sit for centuries undisturbed. We are like that rock. Our potential requires action, it is latent energy waiting to be harnessed. Our job is to give this energy life.

If you attended BJJ classes two times per week consistently for one year that's 104 classes (around 6,240 minutes of BJJ practice). Over the course of ten years that would be 1,040 BJJ classes (62,400 minutes of total BJJ practice). Now if your fellow training partner did the same but tried to train four times per week consistently, they still wouldn't likely achieve better results.

Let's say that they didn't quite train four times per week because they were often injured. Which would more than likely be the case for someone over forty attempting to train this often. It's like the farmer over-fertilizing his fields. More fertilizer won't mean a better crop yield. In fact there may be no crops at all. Overtraining won't get us to our goals quicker.

Small steps over a long haul build mightier bridges. But giant strides that stop short of progress are mostly misguided. Students often think that to be successful in BJJ, they have to make huge, sweeping changes. In fact, steady and consistent efforts, no matter how small, often lead to big, long-lasting results in the long run. The person who starts BJJ and buys three gi's and every piece of gear and trains every day will likely burn out. But the person with one gi who comes to class twice per week without fail will probably achieve more sustainable results. (But never stop short of a few extra gi's)

- The point is that it's okay to have a burst of enthusiasm about starting BJJ (it deserves the attention). But remember success in BJJ doesn't come from owning the fanciest gi or most expensive gear, it's truly time on the mats. As a 40-plus practitioner you can't speed up the progress. You can eliminate barriers to success, but you can't rush the process.

- Just like the farmer who creates the perfect setting for growth, he to cannot hasten its harvest. But he, like you, can slow it down. As a seasoned practitioner your body may not be as resilient as it once was. You may find that recovery takes time and some movements might be more challenging. This should not deter you from training, but rather inspire you to be a wiser, more technical player.

Enjoy all the cool gi's and BJJ gear, but know that nothing can substitute time on the mats. Progress is a bridge that everyone must cross. There's a temptation to look for shortcuts on this journey. You cannot diminish this bridge, but you can make it longer.

Mission:

Focus on structured, incremental learning by mastering the basics. Regularly assess your understanding and skill level through self-reflection and feedback from instructors and peers. Try drills that challenge your adaptability and problem-solving skills like switching between dominant and non-dominant positions and practice escapes from difficult holds to improve both physical and cognitive flexibility. Use techniques such as note-taking, video analysis, and mental rehearsal to deepen your understanding of each move.

Collaborative Learning and Adler

I have found some very interesting parallel's between Alfred Adler's school of psychology and BJJ. Adler believed that a feeling of community and overcoming one's sense of inferiority to strive for personal success were pivotal in an individual's development and psychological well-being. As an older practitioner beginning your BJJ journey you may be reevaluating your own physical and mental identity. This is also true of seasoned practitioners as well. Jiu-Jitsu has a way of continually redefining and then shifting our mind-set.

Adler's school of thought may resonate for you as it offers an interesting blue-print for older grapplers. He believed that an individuals pursuit of excellence is often motivated by a sense of inferiority. As you climb the ladder in BJJ you are like a snake shedding its skin. It is often said that the "real competition is the face looking back at you in the mirror." It's not so much about being better than anyone else. But rather it's about you getting better than your former self.

If you're a new grappler you may experience feelings of inadequacy or doubt. This is normal for anyone starting something new. You're not expected to know what you're doing. In fact embrace this feeling as it will allow you to be a sponge and soak up every detail. This by the way is often the super-power of the seasoned practitioner: the ability to hyper-focus.

With age comes the wisdom of knowing when to pay greater attention to details and understanding the complex connections between moves that can make all the difference. Remember, your brain cannot focus effectively on two things at once. It's like taking a picture with a nice camera. If you focus the camera on an object in the foreground the background becomes blurry (and vice versa). We focus in much the same way. With age and wisdom we know when and where to direct our attention. The younger generation tends to multitask, whereas Gen-X and earlier generations are better at maintaining attention where it's needed. This isn't a knock against the younger generation, as we raised them. With age also comes the humility to learn and the patience to persevere, qualities that are invaluable in the complex world of grappling.

The **inferiority complex** Adler refers to can rear its head for the over 40 practitioner by feeling like you cannot compete with your younger counterparts. The reality is that, like I stated before, the real competition is the face in the mirror. Trying to beat all the young bucks is a fools errand. However this subordinate feeling could have positive aspects as well. It may force you to shift your strategy to relying more on technique and guile and not strength or athleticism. Remember, your wisdom is your strongest asset.

On the other side of the coin we have the opposite of "inferiority" which is a **"superiority" complex** which can be equally challenging. The goal can never be so big that you fail to see the collaborative opportunity you have with your teammates and teachers. Or worse being that person who only cares about themselves and will risk others safety for the "win." When I see someone in my own class going too hard I often joke, "Are you trying to be the champ at Tuesday night 6:00 PM class?" The point is that you have nothing to win and a lot to lose, always put your partners safety first.

It's never black and white like the coin that has superiority on one side and inferiority on the other. Both can be maladaptive ways of approaching Jiu-Jitsu and life. Like most things it's about striking the perfect balance.

Now imagine the coin balanced on its side. By taking a middle road approach you can see and experience the value in both. Where the superiority complex makes it difficult to see the bigger picture, an inferiority complex can amplify feelings of insecurity and doubt. Just like in life we can find a balance of acknowledging our potential for growth while understanding our own unique contributions.

Following a middle ground approach also means that you see the value in other teammates input regarding your training. Remember your training partners are not the competition, but your greatest asset for growth. This doesn't mean you shouldn't have tough, competitive matches. Just be mindful with your own physical boundaries. It's okay to stretch them, just don't break them. The goal is to leave your partners and yourself better than you started.

Here I will share strategies for staying "competitive" with younger, faster, stronger training partners. Remember, technique almost always wins! When you focus on refining every aspect of every technique you can begin to level the playing field. Begin by isolating the four steps to each move and then master them. Once you feel like the four have become one fluid series of movements, add four more steps. When does technique NOT win? When the level of play is equal but one person is stronger, younger and faster, things will change drastically.

It's advantageous to understand their game. One size rarely fits all in clothing or BJJ. You can't apply the same strategy to every match. When you grapple with someone note the patterns and tendencies they follow. Each time try to exploit their game plan. Most people tend to follow a similar path each time they roll. If they are a guard player they'll typically fall backwards. Whereas the passer tends to go to combat base and move forward.

Let's look at specific body styles and physical attributes of others and how we can exploit them for your success.

- **Lanky person** - Their super power is their length. They will be good at maintaining distance and keeping you at bay. You have to treat their legs like two dangerous serpents that can strike and kill you at any moment. If you fall into their guard, maintain a strong posture and keep your neck and arms away from their legs. If you're training with the gi try use your grips to pin their pant legs to the floor. I also find that standing and passing is always a good strategy. Just be mindful of leg entanglements and sweeps when you stand.

- **Lanky person's weaknesses** - It's easier to control longer limbs than shorter ones. They can be more susceptible to joint locks. This includes both upper body (arms) and lower body (leg) attacks. It can also be more difficult to escape moves when you're longer. Smaller bodies tend to get in and out of moves easier. Long limbed practitioners are always dealing with space issues. They tend to get wrapped up easy like a handful of cords tangled in a knot.

- **Lanky person's strengths** - Watch out for triangle chokes, closed guard attacks, hip bump sweeps and leg entanglements. They may be adept at long range sweeps like: double ankle sweep, hook sweep, sickle sweep. The key is to avoid their long legs. But not just the legs as arm triangles, Darce / Anaconda chokes, guillotine chokes can all be dangerous as well!

- **Lanky takedowns** - Watch out for takedowns using their legs like, osotogari and leg trips. A tall person has a leverage advantage and will use takedowns that involve leg to leg and foot trips. In most cases, you won't have to worry about takedowns where their arms are grabbing your legs (double leg, etc.). This is because the knees are a long way down for a taller person which creates greater risks.

- **Big, strong person** - Don't try to match muscle with muscle. In other words don't meet resistance with more resistance. That's not good technique, that's a tug of war. In those situations the younger, stronger person will probably win. Instead meet resistance with opportunities and angles. (In life too) A bigger player will undoubtedly force you to play guard. It's okay to accept guard and then look for a sweep. A sweep can be effective because it requires angular momentum, not strength.

What is angular momentum? -

Think of riding a bike in a straight line. That's linear momentum. Now imagine the bike turns, that's angular momentum. It's like when you spin a top and it continues to keep spinning. Angular momentum is all about the "spin"- how it's created, how much there is and how it can be altered based on how you change the set-up.

Now imagine you're standing in the street and the bike is coming wildly towards you in a straight line (linear momentum). Your options are: to move out of the way, stand there and try to stop it (meeting resistance with resistance), hop on and ride with the momentum, grab on and then create an angle and take it in a different direction (angular momentum). Now think of the bike as a person coming wildly towards you. Your options are the same: to move out of the way, stand there and try to stop them, hop on and ride with the momentum (like a Tomoe-Nage - a circular throw in Judo where you sit back and use your legs to roll them over your head), or grab on to them and create a new angle by moving to the side which is angular momentum. This is a great way to think of how to sweep someone from guard. A sweep is based on three criteria: 1. Disrupt and narrow their base 2. Break their balance, 3. Create an angle and turn their body. With a larger opponent you don't necessarily want to try and trap them inside your guard. They will put pressure on your legs and bulldozer their way through your guard. Instead use your feet on the front of their body to push off them and create distance.

Think of them like a rock wall. You need three points of contact to climb a wall. In order to progress upward at any given time you'll need two feet and one hand connected to the wall. (Or some version) Unless you're Alex Honnold and you can hang from two fingers, normal people always need three points of contact. Apply this same strategy to maintaining your guard.

Having three points of contact from a seated guard position might look like: cross collar grip with your right hand which can be used to pull or push (frame for no-gi), left foot pushing their knee, right foot on the front of their hip to push. The left hand can be a "floater" which can be used to base off the floor or grip and defend when needed.

If you can get a bigger person onto their back you will be in an advantageous position. Like a turtle on its shell, it's harder for a larger person to be mobile from their backside. If you cannot disrupt their base and move them over your body, it might make sense to go underneath them. This can be achieved by using half guard. Butterfly guard is another great way to set up sweeps and go under someone or around them (think of arm drags). One of the big advantages of getting a bigger persons back is you have more coverage area. Whereas a thin person can spin around from the back like a slithering snake, it can be far more difficult for a larger player to escape.

- **Big, strong person's weaknesses** - They will probably move slower and not be as mobile as their smaller counterparts. Bigger grapplers tend to be pressure passers and not typically guard players. If you can get them to their back you have a better opportunity to submit them.

- **Big, strong person's strengths** - The obvious one is that they'll be physically strong. They may have powerful grips and an immoveable base. If they get top position they may make you want to tap from pressure alone. It's very difficult to joint lock really strong players, so look for the choke. It's always the great equalizer for a bigger person.

- **Short, fast and agile person** - The smaller framed agile player has a fair amount of advantages that are unique to this body style. Because they are shorter they have a lower center of gravity. This can make it very difficult to take them down or sweep them from the guard. They also have a higher strength-to-weight ratio. This allows for more explosive movements. For example, bridging to escape from the mount. The compactness of their body and limbs also makes it challenging to submit them. It often seems like the moment you capture their limb, it's gone. You can also forget about triangle chokes too. The only way to capture their limb is to have absolute control of it when attempting a submission.

Think of the arm for a moment. It's made up of three main joints: the shoulder, elbow and the wrist. In order to get a joint lock on a smaller limbed person you need to control two of the three joints at all times. You have to exercise an additional amount of discipline with smaller, agile payers because they can secure dominant position on you quickly. If you go for a submission, make sure you have it.

- **Short, fast and agile person's weaknesses** - While they have many advantages, all body styles and skill-sets have short comings too. Having short limbs means they have limited reach and distance control. It can also be easier to control short legs from the guard. Smaller legs are often easier to get past as you don't deal with length issues. Although they can be harder to leg lock because as you sit back they can pop up easier and also slip out of leg entanglements.

- **Short, fast and agile person's strengths** - Having shorter legs means you can leg pummel more effectively from the guard. Where a longer legged person has to create better angles to slip their legs into triangles from the guard. A smaller legged person can pull their own leg to their chest from the guard and up over their partners shoulders without additional angles. Triangles can be particularly hard for a shorter person to fully lock. However they can use the triangle position to advance into omoplata's. Which I believe is an excellent attack for a short legged player. The omoplata requires a lot of weaving with the legs from tight positions. This falls right into the wheel house for a short person.

If they're fast, don't try and out-speed them, out-wit them. You don't want to sprint with a sprinter. Think for a moment that you're trying to catch a rabbit or a mouse. You would try trap it into a corner and isolate its ability to escape. In the case of a grappling match you need to follow a similar strategy. Don't chase them, corner them by using grips to control their movements.

When you start a match with a fast grappler, immediately establish grips on their sleeve and leg. If it's a no-gi match, try to keep them on their back and control one leg. If you can keep one leg under control and elevated from the floor they can't scramble effectively. If you're trying to advance your position, use your grips to move forward. Always maintain one grip for control as the other hand re-grips. If they're on their back and you're in their guard, start by gripping at the ankle. Next move to the knee, then the hip, etc. never releasing pressure. Don't allow them to escape your physical control. Make it a game of advancing grips.

- **The young wrestler** - Never disregard the power and value of wrestling experience. Even if it was a million years ago and you were in middle school. It's like riding a bike, the skill-set never really goes away. I recently promoted a 55-plus year old to blue belt. He's a smaller guy and hadn't grappled or wrestled since high school. You would be wrong to think that his skill from long ago wouldn't translate into his present experience. But it does. He's very difficult to sweep and his side control is unforgivable.

- However, he was always easy to triangle and guillotine. Why would I say those two submissions? Because wrestlers tend to lead with their head, which leaves their neck exposed. Just like you can't beat the sprinter by sprinting. Neither should you attempt to beat the wrestler by wrestling with them. They are going to to be naturally strong scramblers. Which means they can often control quick unpredictable situations. It's far better to use their power and energy against them and play the long game, while looking for their mistakes.

- **Strategic adaptation** is an important principle to apply to your BJJ practice. This refers to the ability to modify and adapt your techniques to a rapidly changing environment. This can be particularly effective with wrestlers who can force a scramble. By learning to 'go with the flow' of the match you can better harness your energy and use a wrestler's own strength and momentum against them. This idea of using opponent's energy against is a cornerstone of BJJ.

- **The young wrestlers strengths** - Fast, explosive and effective at creating and controlling scrambles. They often have good cardio, but not in all cases. If you have someone who may have wrestled years ago but their current cardio doesn't match their experience, it may work against them. Wrestlers tend to rely on what they know best. If they are in "less than ideal" shape they may tire quickly. They are also very difficult to take down or sweep from the guard.

- **The young wrestlers weaknesses** - They will often lead with their head which leaves them open for strangles. (Triangle chokes, loop chokes and guillotines are all "kryptonite" for wrestlers) As previously mentioned they may have poor cardio from a lack of training they might also revert back to wrestling and tire quickly.

Know that every grappling match is an opportunity for growth, expansion and collaboration. Beyond the technical aspects and strategies lies a journey of personal growth that transcends the mats. By pushing each other in training we prepare ourselves for the real world where resilience and mental toughness are often the antidotes for stress and anxiety. Have you heard the saying, "Embrace the suck"? Yes, but also embrace the "push."

Start by recognizing the unique gift our body offers to Jiu-Jitsu. Every body style has both positive and negative attributes. By understanding where our strengths lie and weakness reveal themselves we only become better. Review the list of body styles and see where your own strengths and weaknesses are and how you can strengthen them. In addition, you can begin to strategize for partners you may face on the mats. How can you adapt your game when needed and take advantage of your partners weaknesses. See where you can apply strategic adaptation to your game. Look for partners in your academy that fit these physical attributes and apply new strategies to your matches with them.

Finally, see the importance of collaboration in your Jiu-Jitsu experience. How can you grow with your partners and not against them. If you share with your partners where they are making mistakes, instead of just repeatedly capitalizing on them, you both get better.

Visualization

People train BJJ for a variety of reasons: competition, exercise, social connections, self-defense, etc. You probably didn't start BJJ so you could beat the crap out of the wiry young lions that train in your dojo. If you make that your focus (and it does sound fun from time to time) you will probably end up on the bench. If you feel like you need to prove something? Well you don't, because you did already by starting your training in BJJ and not quitting.

The best piece of advice I have heard for rolling is to *"not try to win in practice."* Instead of making everything a competition, embrace a learning mindset. Focus your energy on expanding your knowledge base and BJJ comprehension. Every roll offers a greater lesson. Take copious mental notes on each grappling match. Note how you feel, but also your mindset.

Did you feel calm and controlled or were you frustrated and unfocused? Don't avoid challenges, embrace them as an opportunity for growth. This doesn't mean to push yourself through physical pain. But yes, often times you do need to go beyond the mental pain.

Ask yourself:

"Do I have mental lapses when I am rolling that cause me to lose positions, techniques and opportunities?"

"Do I just give up sometimes, do I quit?"

I have answered yes to both of these questions. Everyone is going to lose focus and give up at times. This is the harsh reality that we all face in the practice of this unforgiving art. You can't lie to Jiu-Jitsu, she will call you on it every single time. You can kid yourself and say that you were tired or they were bigger or faster or whatever. Sometimes those may be factored into the equation. But if you know in your heart that sometimes you just quit, then it's time to forge a new path.

Start be embracing the fact that BJJ is a tough sport and requires resilience. Nobody is born resilient, it is earned mostly through overcoming hardship. It's like building callous's on your feet. When people first start BJJ with me I often joke that they have "Bambi feet." Meaning they'll get terrible mat burn, until they don't. The toughness has to be earned, it doesn't come in a day.

So if you don't feel that "toughness" yet that's okay, just keep coming. Attending class on the days you don't feel like it is one of the best ways to flex your discipline muscles. Even if you have to drag your bag behind you as you begrudgingly walk through the doors. This is how you build grit. Not the outdated, old model of the "No pain no gain mentality." But rather maintaining a positive mental attitude in the face of obstacles.

One of my favorite mantras is: "I act in spite of inconvenience, I act in spite of fear, I act in spite of obstacles." By moving forward and facing what makes you uncomfortable you build confidence. Conquering your fears, doubts and anxieties prepares you to deal with future challenges (on and off the mats).

BJJ Visualization techniques - Visualization is a powerful tool to help you enhance your performance on the mats. By mentally rehearsing your outcome you can pre-pave a successful path. When you visualize a grappling scenario your brain activates many of the same neural pathways as when you physically perform it. This strengthens the neural connections and makes it easier to draw upon the techniques later. Better retention of techniques makes it easier to develop adaptability and muscle memory when you're live rolling and things change rapidly.

Find yourself a quiet space where you won't be interrupted. You can use your meditation time for mental rehearsal as well. Close your eyes and picture a blank movie screen in front of you. You are both the director, screen writer and main star of this film. This means that you get to control the flow and outcome. Start by seeing yourself in your BJJ training gear and you're calm, cool and collected. Your face is relaxed, your body is free from tension. As you breathe slowly, release any tension from your face.

Now breathe in and out and relax your entire body from the top of your head to the bottom of your toes. Slowly breathe in and breathe out any tension.

Now that you're relaxed, begin to create the movie masterpiece of your grappling. You can envision new matches of yourself moving flawlessly from sweep to submission. Or you can reflect on previous experiences where you struggled and now you create a new storyline.

Visualize areas of your grappling that are weak and need attention. Create scenarios where you no longer struggle in those positions but have a positive experience. This will set the tone for when you face these "real world" challenges in the future. Your body won't react in fear, but rather with confidence and a sense of familiarity.

Imagine yourself in what would normally be a "bad" position for you. But instead you're in control and masterfully reverse the position. Remember, this is your story and you get to create the perfect ending that serves you best. (Spoiler alert - you're the hero in this narrative) When you combine mental practice with physical reps you can get even more profound results.

Tips for combining mental and physical practice:

We have also included BJJ affirmations that can help guide you towards a positive outcome. With affirmations use 'present-tense' language, speak in a positive tone, and practice often.

Pre-competition visualization - If you're a competitor or aspiring competitor this is a great way to pre-pave your results. Spend some time before the event mentally rehearsing your successful outcome. See yourself calmly responding under pressure with ease and fluidity. Build details into the storyline. Picture yourself on the awards stand and feel the weight of the gold medal hanging around your neck. Feel the emotions. Activate all your senses.

Pre-competition affirmations -

"I am confident and prepared for this competition"

"I move with ease and fluidity. Everything is there when I need it"

"I am on top, tuned up and ready to go!"

"I release all fear and anxiety and embrace the present moment"

"I trust in my ability to make lightning fast decisions that serve my game"

These can be done daily, in a quiet space, leading up to the event. You can also use them as quick triggers right before you compete. Here are some competition mental cues that work well.

As you bow onto the mats to compete say to yourself,

"I am confident and ready!"

"It's my time"

"I am confident and in control"

"I embrace the challenge"

"I've got this"

"The work is done, let's go!"

Pre-Class visualization -

It's totally normal to have anxiety around going to BJJ class. This doesn't make you weak. It's very common and manageable. Remind yourself that the more you attend classes, the less stress you will feel. Consistency will breed familiarity which in turn builds self-confidence. When you arrive to class try to spend a few minutes in your car visualizing. Mentally rehearse yourself confidently and assuredly entering the school. Picture yourself having a great class where you are having fun overcoming challenges.

Pre-class affirmations -

"My knowledge and skills improve with every class I attend"

"I value the opportunity to absorb BJJ wisdom and knowledge"

"My age is my super power, I bring wisdom and insight"

"My body is strong and supports my BJJ training"

"I am flexible in my thoughts and actions"

"I belong here and bring value to my teammates"

Mental cues for when you're in class - Remember the goal is to shift focus towards something positive. You're going to have moments of doubt and insecurity when you're in class. When negativity creeps in say to yourself, "This thought holds no power, I'm in control."

"Trust in the process"

"Breathe out the doubt"

"Keep going"

"I've got this"

"Stay focused"

"Stay in the present"

"Be patient"

"Breathe"

"Progress not perfection"

"I'm better with every breath"

"I'm having fun challenging myself"

"All is well"

Technical visualization -

This is where you take complete command over your motor skills and performance of a technique. Notice how I said "performance." The goal isn't just to be good with a move but to develop mastery with it. To be able to call upon the technique without hesitation and execute it flawlessly. This is where you can now perform the move for your audience (your partner in this case). Except they won't be applauding, but hopefully tapping.

With technical visualization you want to focus on mastering the four steps of each move. Picture yourself, and feel yourself performing the technique. See it both from a third person perspective (like seeing yourself in a movie). But also from your own point of view as if you were seeing it through your own eyes as you do it.

You can also combine the physical repetitions with mental reps. Start by physically performing the four steps of the move on your partner. Stop at certain points and either mentally or verbally state the next series of steps. Stating them without physical movement forces you to create a stronger mental image of the move.

Recovery and Recuperation visualization -

This is where you consciously work on your breathing and visualization techniques guided towards an active recovery.

Body scanning technique -

Using this form of guided imagery you can examine your entire body and zero in on specific sources of discomfort or pain. If you do this on a regular basis you can develop a deep mind and body connection. You will be able to detect "warning signs" in your body earlier.

Visualization script -

Close your eyes, take a deep breath. Imagine a warm ray of light emanating from the crown of your head. Pull the light down and imagine it slowly traveling down through your body and scanning every inch. Picture each body part being warmed by the light. Connect your thoughts to your breath. If you feel any pain or discomfort, spend a moment breathing and relaxing that area. The goal is to scan your entire body from top to bottom.

Injury prevention script -

Imagine that you're in your academy in your full gear (gi or no-gi) and you're training with a partner. Picture yourself in a grappling match and things suddenly go wrong. Maybe you twist your knee as you defend a move. Breathe deep and stay relaxed as you picture yourself reacting. You are calm and your leg turns in the perfect direction relieving any tension and keeping you safe. You feel strong, supported and flexible. It feels good to train safely.

Healing and recovery script -

If you're currently dealing with an injury this can be helpful. Close your eyes and breathe deeply from your belly. Now visualize your inured body part. Imagine it being engulfed in a warm light. Picture the healing happening as your blood carries nutrients to your injured body part. See the inflammation reducing and the tissue rebuilding itself as the pain slowly slips away. Feel the strength in your body as you breathe out any pain.

With any injury it is important to see a medical professional right away and get a proper diagnosis, not from me, or your buddies on the mat! I can break you, but I can't fix you!

Mission:

With this operation we went deep down the rabbit hole of mental Jiu-Jitsu. We started out discussing imposter syndrome. If you're grappling with feelings of not deserving your rank or stagnation in progress, it's often a case of how you perceive things. Perception often becomes reality. When your children are toddlers, you don't really notice them getting bigger and taller. But then one day it hits you and you see the progression all at once.

Evolution on the mats happens over time but is generally recognized in retrospect. Much like watching children grow, improvements in your skills and abilities on the mats occur gradually and often subtly. Day-to-day, it might be hard to notice the small increments of change, but over time, these small improvements accumulate.

It's important to remember that progress isn't always linear, it generally follows a curved trajectory.

Utilize the list of goals and accompanying affirmations to help get you over your own mental hurdles. You can also write out your goals in your BJJ notebook with supportive affirmations. Find the ones that resonate most with you.

Update all of your goals regularly with new affirmations to support them. If for example your goal is to get your purple belt injury-free. The supporting affirmation might sound like, "I am committed to staying injury free on my road to purple!" If you need some motivation and inspiration, look no further than the reflection cast in your mirror. BJJ is a tough journey and your resilience to continue should be commended.

Look for opportunities to celebrate the small victories along the way.

"The Specialist" Versus "The Generalist"

In the context of medicine a generalist can treat a wide range of health challenges. Whereas a specialist may have expertise in a more narrow range of skills. There is value in both depending on your goals and where you are in your training. In the framework of BJJ a new white belt may be learning a wider range of new moves. Mostly because as a novice, everything is new. A purple or brown belt on the other hand may be honing and mastering a very specific game. For example, they might wear a purple belt, but have a brown belt skill-set at their speciality. I can relate to this as a black belt. My "specialty" is the triangle choke. I feel that my skillset matches my belt rank. Can I say that about every move, of course not. The difference as a black belt professor is that I can teach just about any move. But that comes from understanding the BJJ framework. A good teacher is both a specialist and a generalist.

You don't need to be good at everything. But if you truly understand the BJJ framework you can teach just about anything. This is why black belts become "**professors**." The word *professor means, teacher.*

"To teach is to learn." When you teach a BJJ technique to someone else, you have to break it down into smaller parts, explain it in a way that the other person can understand, and often adjust and adapt the technique based on how well the student can perform it. This forces you to truly know the move.

Specialist - They have honed a specific set of movements and can guide a match towards their desired position or preferred sequences. Whereas the generalist doesn't limit their game to one single position. I think ultimately a combination of both is the best strategy. You may want to develop an ever-evolving game, but have your "go-to" when you need it. It's vital to be good at a lot of things, but have a deep level of mastery with one or two specific areas. Like with the Pareto principle, or 80/20 rule, the majority of our BJJ success will come from a very small set of moves. It won't always be divided as 80/20 either. In reality you might hit 65% of your sweeps, for example, from 25% of your moves. The math isn't as important as recognizing that you don't need to know everything. But you should at least have a vague understanding of most things. You might not be good at triangles, but others will try to submit you with them. Therefore, you at least need to know the basics of the triangle attack.

Below are examples of positional specialists -

Bottom control (Guard position) -

Closed guard / open guard

Half guard

Deep half guard

K-guard

Z-guard

Lasso guard

Inverted guard

High guard

Spider guard

Knee shield

X-guard

De La Riva / reverse

Butterfly guard

Rubber guard

Worm guard

Donkey guard

Collar sleeve guard

Seated guard

William's guard

50/50 guard

Top Control (Mount / Side / Back) -

S-mount

Traditional side control (100 kilos)

Scarf hold (Kesa gatame)

Reverse scarf hold (facing opponents legs with the arm trapped)

Twister side control (facing the legs, but with no arm trapped)

North / south

Knee on belly

Full mount

Leg lock / Leg entanglement specialist -

Ashi-garami

Outside Ashi-garami

Inside Ashi-garami

Honey hole

411

Saddle

Ankle lace

Inside Sankaku

Single leg X-guard

50/50

Many of these positions are subsets or variants of other positions.

Below are examples of submission specialists -

Arm lock

Darce choke

Wrist lock

Omoplata

Triangle choke

Kimura lock

Leg locks

Lapel chokes

Back specialist

Choke - RNC Rear Naked Choke, gi / lapel / collar chokes, etc.

Ezekiel choke

In some cases you may have a combination of submissions that you are most adept at executing. For example the triangle choke and omoplata. Since both attacks are always within the same vicinity, they tend to go hand in hand. My professor always referred to them as "brother and sister."

Where there is one, you'll almost always find the other attack nearby. This is also true of the triangle choke and the straight armlock.

How do you decide what you will specialize in? This often comes down to a combination of factors. First and foremost you'll most certainly be influenced by your professor's own stylistic preferences. If they're a "triangler," that essence will rub off on their students. Next you will likely gravitate to moves that match your body style and physical attributes. If you are long and lean you might find that triangles fit nicely into your game. On the flip side, if you're short and stocky, half guard might be your cup of tea.

Of course moves can cross over between body styles. In addition, your own personality may come into play. If you tend to be more of a 'control freak' you may want to create a flow chart and specific strategies. If you are more of a 'risk taker' you may gravitate to a more conceptual game. One that allows you the freedom to "fly by the seat of your pants." These ideologies will most likely shift as you evolve in your game and as you age.

When I was a younger (and lower ranked) practitioner my game was very much fast and athletic and relied more on my instincts than a game plan. As I've "matured" in my practice (and my age) I have found that slowing things down and having a game plan most often serves me (and my body) best.

Below we have matched body styles to specific attacks and submissions. These are just examples of attacks and positions. Feel free to add even more that fit into your personal game.

Flexible body

Advantages - They can transition their legs without having to shrimp their hips. This also allows for better escapes, attacks and sweeps.

Type of attacks - Triangle chokes, gogoplata, omoplata, berimbolos, ezekiels.

Positions - Rubber guard, open guard, spider guard, lasso guard, *inverted guard, high guard, William's guard, Granby rolls, 50/50.

Small framed body

Advantages - They can escape moves easier. Their smaller limbs are more difficult to control and submit.

Types of attacks - Triangle choke, omoplata, armbars, sweeps, lapel chokes, leg locks.

Positions - Half guard, deep half guard, closed guard, high guard, butterfly guard, x-guard, back takes, lapel guard, 50/50.

Long and lean

Types of attacks - Triangle choke, arm triangle, anaconda choke, Darce choke, omoplata, leg entanglements, cryangle choke, ezekiel, and leg locks.

Positions - Lasso guard, lapel guard, full guard, worm guard, spider guard, high guard, William's guard, body triangle, s-mount, 50/50, De La Riva guard.

Strong body type

Types of attacks - Kimura, americana, North / south choke, rear naked choke, collar chokes, guillotine choke, head and arm choke (arm triangle), Ezekiel, "Mother's milk."

Positions - Takedowns, side control, kesa gatame, pressure passing, mount, s-mount, butterfly guard, body triangle.

Short and stocky

Advantages - Shorter limbs are more difficult to control and submit. They have a lower center of gravity which makes them harder to sweep. But also gives them the upper hand on take downs and takedown defense.

Types of attacks - Kimura, americana, guillotine choke, head and arm chokes (arm triangle), omoplata.

Positions - Butterfly guard, half guard, deep half guard, full guard - over and under hooks, pressure passing, side control attacks, knee on the belly, kesa gatame.

Short legs

Advantages - Their smaller frame and shorter legs allows them to get under their opponents and load their weight more effectively. This is particularly helpful in setting up sweeps, executing back takes and leg attacks. They can also enter smaller spaces more efficiently and with better results.

Types of attacks - Kimura, americana, rear naked choke, armbars (top, bottom and side), gi / no-gi back chokes and armbars (from the back), leg locks.

Positions - Take downs (lower center of gravity), duck under, butterfly guard, knee on the belly, north south, back takes, pressure passing.

Fast and athletic

Advantages - They can advance quickly from position to position with little recovery. They can often execute more dynamic moves and difficult transitions.

Types of attacks - Knee slice passes, athletic passes, quick back takes (chokes), Darce choke, triangle choke, leg locks.

Positions - Scrambling, *inverted guard, berimbolo, *jumping / flying techniques, guard passing, take downs.

Large frame

Advantages - They are able to apply "tap inducing" side control pressure. In addition they may also have significant mount control as well. This will lead to more submission opportunities as they can control and tire their opponents.

Types of attacks - Ezekiel, kimura, head and arm choke (arm triangle), cross collar choke, lapel chokes, americana, guillotine choke, north south choke, "Mother's milk."

Positions - Side control, north south, mount.

This is a fun way to consider other positions and attacks. We gave you a guideline, but you can continue to expand this into your own BJJ eco system. With the advent of companies like "BJJ Fanatics" you can study instructional courses from various teachers that match your body style. I have found that in my own instructional courses I like to teach in a way that addresses and makes accommodations for all body styles. If you're a professor or hope to be one some day, I recommend adopting this inclusive teaching style into your practice.

Mission:

Try out a few different visualizations and guided meditations we've included in this book. Write some of your favorite affirmations and be sure to memorize a few for when you're in class too.

Write out your four steps to a technique in your BJJ notebook. Read it aloud repeatedly until you have it memorized. Shorten the steps if needed. We refer to this as "technical visualization." The objective is to internalize the move without moving your body. You can use it for injury prevention, recovery, anxiety, pre-comp jitters, body scanning / awareness and more. Play audio from visualizations as you drive to class. Think of it as a mental warm up.

Do your own research on some of the "brain supplements" we've listed. Apply the DTP formula; or demonstrate, teach and perform. The further you go into a technique, the quicker it becomes a part of you. This is quite literally true as we discussed with the concept of "neuroplasticity" or the brains ability to alter and reorganize its structure based on new experiences. Remember, teaching leads to faster assimilation.

Who are you teaching? Yourself! You can video record yourself at home doing a move (demonstration). As you demonstrate the move, speak the four steps aloud as you do them. Execute it 3-4 times during the recording. This gives you a larger sample size. You then review the video frame by frame to evaluate your own technique. Look for consistency, accuracy of the steps and fluidity. Ideally the performance aspect is you doing it correctly during a live roll. Try it on someone less skilled than you, so you have a better chance at success. Record yourself doing your reps for 2-3 minutes without a rest on a grappling dummy at home. This is a great way to build consistency, accuracy and fluidity in your execution of the technique without a live partner.

Do the drills we've included to understand principle versus conceptual based learning. Begin to apply these ideas into your own BJJ game. If you're a teacher or coach, these drills can be very effective for your students. Begin to consider new positions that you're not familiar with practicing or teaching. Try to view them from both an offensive (you're attacking) and defensive perspective. You can research these positions on YouTube to further your understanding.

Acquaint yourself with matching attacks to body styles. This will give you a better understanding of what you'll be facing on the mats and why. Find your own body style and attacks that work best with it. As a teacher, it's important to understand how body styles match up to specific techniques. This gives you a much larger framework to teach from that addresses the individual needs of your students.

Debriefing Assessment:

Blending the sharpness of your mind with the strength of your body isn't just helpful in Brazilian Jiu-Jitsu—it's crucial. We've explored how adopting a robust philosophy can elevate your practice, connecting every physical move with a mental strategy. Remember our discussion on jotting down key moves and discovering a learning style that resonates with you? That's your solid base to build upon.

We also tackled some real game-changers for keeping your mental game strong. Think about those tips for boosting your memory—like optimizing your diet and employing smart, brain-boosting strategies. And let's not overlook the inner battles, like taking on Imposter Syndrome and recognizing when the Dunning-Kruger effect might be skewing your self-perception. It's all about gaining deeper self-awareness, right?

We balanced these deeper insights with practical ways to apply both principles and concepts in your training—keeping it real on the mats as we do in our discussions. And how about that team vibe from our collaborative learning session? Plus, flexing your mental muscles with visualization and deciding whether you're more of a Specialist or a Generalist—each approach has its unique strengths.

All of this is about setting you up not just to succeed, but to excel, making every session meaningful and every technique impactful.

Survival Expert:
BRENT BURNISTON

---

age 47, Brazilian Jiu-Jitsu, 4th Degree Black Belt
Founder and Owner of Subconscious Jiu-Jitsu Academy
Co-Founder of Subconscious Jiu-Jitsu Association
Lineage: Jean Jacques Machado / Roger Gracie (currently)

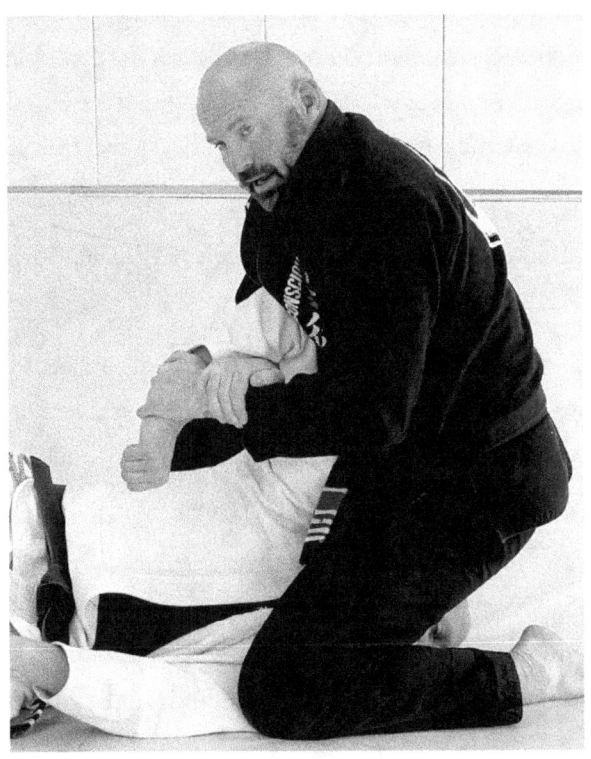

Intel:

Growing up Brent's father was a 6-time Golden Gloves Champion and a wellrespected boxing coach in the Midwest. So, he spent a lot of time with his father at the Fort Wayne PAL boxing club. At age 6 his mother enrolled him in Judo hoping he'd do that instead of getting in a ring and fighting like his father. He continued to train in the martial arts: Judo, Karate, and Boxing with his dad throughout his childhood. Being a huge Bruce Lee fan, he was influenced with the ideas in Lee's book, the Tao of Jeet Kune Do. It was really in that book that gave exposure to the idea of mixed martial arts that got him hooked. He would practice with his friend and first ever training partner Lane Andrews (also now a Robson Moura Black Belt) in their garage.

Then in November of 1993, while at a friend's house flipping channels, they see the Ultimate Fight Championship. Neither could believe it!! A skinny Brazilian guy strangled everyone and won the championship. Brent knew at that point he needed to learn Brazilian Jiu-Jitsu. He started attending all the Royce Gracie seminars in the Midwest and training with early MMA fighters.

After graduating Brent moved to Los Angeles to pursue his dream of becoming a black belt in Jiu-Jitsu.

Though a successful competitor during his early days, Brent was forced to put competition on hold as he was hired on as a world leader in executive protection. With almost 20 years of experience, Brent has led multi-man protective details spanning the globe.

As one of Jean Jacques Machado's top students and instructors Brent received his Black Belt in 2009. In 2010 Brent established Subconscious Jiu-Jitsu Academy in North Hollywood. In 2021 Brent co-founded Subconscious Jiu-Jitsu Association, with friend and training partner Nic Gregoriades.

From the Source:

During my Senior year of football, I sustained a major injury to my neck after getting tackled. I rolled my neck so far under me that my opposite ear ended up touching the ground. The injury caused me to have to have two "S" shape curvatures to my spine, I twisted my pelvis, and caused my coccyx to dislocate. I was rushed to the hospital where doctors were convinced, I broke my neck because of all the trauma to my spine. After (3) MRI's they were unable to find a break to all their amazement. After some physical therapy I went on to play three years of D1 College Football before the injury ultimately forced me to give it up for good.

Even though the neck injury forced me to give up football, I was still very active practicing Jiu-Jitsu, wrestling, and kickboxing. With these sports it always seemed like I was able to brace myself or protect my neck in ways that I just couldn't in football. I found ways to avoid my neck being cranked on or injuring it. Even to this day (because of this early emphasis on protecting my neck) I don't expose my neck very often and almost never find myself in a bad position that my neck is in danger. I've just put so much focus on keeping my neck safe for all these years that I've trained myself not to expose it where someone can injure me.

This injury really taught me that even if you have some limitations, you can almost always still train around them. Sometimes these limitations may even become strengths. Train smart and know your limits and make sure to let your training partners know your injuries before they crank on them. Don't ever be ashamed to tap when you find yourself in a bad position.

- **My advice is always start slow.** You don't need to spar 4-5 times a week when you're first starting out. I recommend you attend 3-4 classes a week, but spar (high intensity) no more than twice for the first few weeks. (Depending on your physical shape it may be zero times starting off.) I like to tell my older beginners to never spar two days in a row either. Always allow a day or two between hard rolls until you condition yourself to be able to pick up the intensity.

- The days you do spar I would recommend focusing more of your training on **CONTROL** and **DEFENSE**. As an older grappler it's taxing on us to try and go out and chase submissions the whole round. Instead look for ways to get to your favorite positions or positions you have the most success at and spend a lot of time trying to maintain that position. Learn two or three submissions or sweeps from there. The more you put yourself in these positions of advantage the more likely you're going to find success and waste a lot less energy. AND ALWAYS REMEMBER. *You don't need to be better than someone in Jiu-Jitsu, you just need to be better than them in a particular position that you can put them.* If I'm going to get beat, I want to be beat where my Jiu-Jitsu is strongest. Where I am the most comfortable. If you beat me at my own game, fair play. You were better than me at my Jiu-Jitsu today. But if I allow you to put me in your favorite position(s) I'm already way behind the 8 ball and likely will spend a lot of energy trying to escape those positions and ultimately most likely tapping.

Number 1 survival tip:

Train as though It's a marathon, not a sprint. It's about consistency and keeping yourself free from injuries as much as you can.

A few of the ways I stay healthy off the mats:

- Ice or cold bath on training days
- Everyday Jiu-Jitsu specific supplements (Fish oil, glucosamine, Joint Supplement, magnesium, Zinc, Cordyceps mushrooms, Organic Turkey Tail mushrooms, Creatine, and protein powder)
- Stretching before and after workouts.

- I don't spar hard two days in a row anymore. It's better to spar every other day and be on the mat 5-6 days than kill yourself twice a week.

- If / when I lift weights, I lift to prevent injury, and gain conditioning /endurance. Lighter weight, higher reps. I also usually stay away from dips and other exercises that put extra tension on my knees and elbows. Jiu-Jitsu does enough of that. (I have horrible knees and elbows)

- I'd be lying if I said I had the best diet, but I do my best to try to eat mostly carnivore with fruits, and honey Monday-Friday. I usually cheat more on the weekends. I almost always avoid gluten, wheat, soy, and flour and anything inflammatory. Avoiding those four things has helped my joint pain probably more than probably anything else.

- Massage 1-2 times a month and see a physical therapist / chiropractor 2-3 times a month if you have the funds.

- My number one advice to my younger self or anyone starting out in BJJ is **take care of your injuries when they happen.** If you're injured take time off and heal them properly. Do the physical therapy, and be good to your body especially your knees, elbows, and shoulders. You've only got one body, so take care of it and make it last.

I've been doing Jiu-Jitsu now for more than 25 years so I can't say I have too many unexpected benefits, however I'm still surprised at how much I still yearn to be a student even after all these years. I would've thought at this point I'd have a pretty good grasp of Jiu-Jitsu and maybe won't have the same desire to train / learn. But that's simply just not the case. I'm still learning so much these days, maybe even more now then ever before! With the online sites, books, YouTube, etc., there is so much information out there. I think this constant chase of self-improvement and drive for excellence bleeds into many areas of my life that maybe I wouldn't have thought would.

I live and approach life through Jiu-Jitsu and because of that I'm a better human in my 40's and hopefully even better in my close approaching 50's.

Without a doubt the thing that inspires me most these days are my students. Teaching Jiu-Jitsu and watching my students progress brings me as much joy as any achievements I could personally earn. With that being said, I still really enjoy learning and refining my own Jiu-Jitsu game as well. Every few months I get the chance to spend some time on the mat with someone like Roger Gracie and I always walk away thinking I don't know anything about Jiu-Jitsu. These training days remind me that I still have so much more to learn and refine. Jiu-Jitsu is truly a lifelong study and something very few will ever master, and this motivates me like few things do and because of that I don't see myself giving up anytime soon! Hopefully (Jiu-Jitsu Gods willing) I'll continue to ride this train until the wheels fall completely off.

Operations:

Embrace Technology

Advice on leveraging technology for learning and improving BJJ skills, with a focus on apps, online resources, and virtual reality training possibilities.

Scan the QR code for tutorials on video analysis, home training setups, and more.

https://www.youtube.com/playlist?list=PLwb5iQup9939Iu
YLOlZQu60vX5mWSR6zC

Hacking Everything Tech

We live in an age where technology can be used to improve our training dramatically. If you're over 40 like me, you may come from the old school. You may not be a "tech-head." But by embracing current technology you can greatly enhance your BJJ experience.

If seeing and hearing yourself on video makes you squirm, don't worry you're not alone. As someone who has put out thousands of online tutorials, I hated seeing myself on video at first. I cringed watching myself move and hearing myself speak. It took me some time to get comfortable with the experience. Now after several years watching and editing myself, I can see the value in it. Many people share this same anxiety.

Since we only see certain angles of our own face in the mirror, it can seem strange to see ourselves as others see us. This heightened sense of self-awareness can cause us to be hyper-aware of certain flaws, quirks and mannerisms. Over time you will become more comfortable with observing yourself. Don't miss out on this opportunity. In psychology they call this phenomenon the "familiarity principle." It says that the more we are exposed to something the more we prefer it.

It's helpful to get comfortable with understanding your own body mechanics and the way you move in different environments against different opponents. By consistently observing and analyzing your BJJ mechanics, reactions, and habits, you'll develop a deeper connection within yourself.

Not only will you understand your own strengths and weaknesses, you'll develop a sense of holistic (whole body) awareness. To have the ability to observe my own technique from a third person perspective has been invaluable. By studying my own mechanical tendencies I have gained the ability to "edit" and revise my own technique.

We operate in world where we have amazing high quality video in the palm of our hands. It's not like the old days when we had to lug that huge Sony VHS camera onto our shoulder. When you video yourself try to get a mix of matches from different levels. This will give you a wider perspective to evaluate from. Try to spot your mistakes and note where you could make changes. If you get submitted attempt to retrace your steps in the video. If for example you got arm-barred from mount, look back and re-examine the 4 - 5 steps that precipitated the submission. Remember, it's never one thing that happened. It's almost always an avalanche of errors. Try to determine what lead to the "disaster."

- A grappling dummy can be an excellent tool for videoing your execution of techniques. There's a lot of options for training dummies online. If you're uncomfortable videoing yourself with live partners, this can be a great alternative. Simply set up your smart phone on a tripod and video yourself performing techniques in the safety and comfort of your garage or basement.

- If you have the space and budget, it can be worth adding a small matted training area at home. Mats can be purchased fairly inexpensively online depending on the quality. There's everything from cheap puzzle mats (which can work well), to folding gymnastics mats, to more expensive and intricate systems. A small matted area can also work great if you want to invite teammates over for additional training.

In some cases where you don't have an academy near you this can be a workable alternative. If this is your situation, you might be able to find training partners or other BJJ enthusiasts in your area. I've heard of people starting a training group like this that evolved into something more substantial. In fact one gentleman I spoke to started a training meet-up out of his basement and eventually attracted a brown belt who began teaching the group. If you build it, they might just come!

If you have the space for home training I recommend going for it. If you can video yourself with a live partner or grappling dummy, you can compare your technique to high-level practitioners you admire. You can search out YouTube videos of them teaching or competing and make comparisons. If you like to utilize online tutorials you can compare your technique to the teacher you're studying. This will help you see how the move looks when done correctly and help you identify any adjustments needed.

Regularly recording yourself grappling with a partner will help you track your progress in real-time. This can be a great confidence boost as well! It's important to watch your videoed sessions over and over again. This is form of mental rehearsal. By viewing yourself doing the move, you can create a feedback-loop that tells your brain, this is how it's done correctly.

Welcome to the Future:

In this section I'll share several ways to utilize video to elevate your training. If you're a visual, reading / writing or auditory leaner, you may align perfectly with video as a learning tool. Don't worry kinesthetic learners, we will cross that bridge together too. Here we will match each learning style with its own 'best practices' for using video for performance enhancement.

Visual Learners

They learn the best by seeing *images* and *drawings*. Visual learners do well with reviewing techniques through video. You can record yourself performing a technique while audibly speaking each step. You can do *mental reps* later at your convenience from anywhere you can use your phone. This is the luxury of video, you have a perfect archival record for later. Watch the video over and over with the volume turned up and also with no sound at all.

You can also take a screen shot of each important step of the move. You can then physically draw on the images and add additional notes. Another option for visual learners is to record your rolling sessions and review it on pause while advancing it frame by frame. This will allow you to deeply analyze each movement, transition, and response close up.

You've heard of the saying, "The devil is in the details." I say, "The success is in the details!" Often the difference between a technique working and not is the small, minute components.

When you watch a match frame by frame, you'll be able to identify the precise moments where adjustments are needed. You'll also see where your tendencies and habits are and if they support a positive outcome.

Once you identify your areas of improvement you can begin to visualize the correct responses by mentally rehearsing them. Match analysis will also provide insights into better strategizing during your rounds. As you observe your grappling look for patterns and tendencies in both your own movements and those of your opponents. What do your transitions *look* like? Are they smooth and efficient, or are they slow and clunky? Are you staying focused and in the zone? Or do you experience lapses in defense that leave you vulnerable?

Recording your training sessions is a great instrument for learning. You can set up your phone propped against a wall when you're rolling. As a show of good etiquette be sure to tell your partners in advance that you're videoing them. Let them know it's only for private consumption and for learning. Never post your private grappling matches on social media. In my opinion, rolling is a private affair and should not be shared in that way.

You could even sit after the roll and review the video together. This is a great way to collaborate and share insights.

Auditory Learners

They benefit from hearing and speaking in learning environments. When you record yourself performing a move on a live partner or grappling dummy, audibly speak the steps aloud. You can then play back the audio while you practice the moves on a partner or dummy. Hearing your own voice will reinforce the steps in your mind and provide a rhythm to the sequence of the movements.

For example: If you're doing an a triangle choke, play the audio from the video in the background and follow along to your narration. Hearing your own voice can tap into your own natural preference of auditory learning. Your brain will instantly 'turn on' with the sound of your own voice guiding the way.

Auditory learners also do well with affirmations. You can add positive self-talk or motivational cues alongside the technical instructions when recording your sessions. This not only reinforces the techniques but also boosts your confidence and mindset during practice. Instead of just speaking the four steps to an armbar in a non-emotional mechanical way, you can add depth to the technique that will resonate with you.

For example with the armbar from the mount:

1. Replace "grab the arm at the shoulder and elevate it" with "I confidently secure my partners arm at the shoulder"

2. Replace "Post the opposite leg and slide the near side leg under their head" with "I post my opposite leg as I fluidly rotate my hips and slide my near side leg tightly under their head"

3. Replace "Post on their head and bring my leg over their head" with

"I keep my hips low barely hovering over their body as I slide my leg over their head to be sure to cover every aspect of their body like a shadow"

4. Replace "Lie back and squeeze the legs together as the hips are elevated" with "I lay my body backwards and pinch my knees tightly together as I confidently control all three joints on their arm confidently securing the submission"

The difference in the second example is that I am using a first person perspective (I, me, my versus impersonal language cues). This will help strengthen the cognitive function by making it personal, memorable and powerful.

When you're learning new techniques, whether from in a classroom or an online tutorial, your brain will better assimilate the new knowledge by hearing your own voice. When you're learning from online courses you can also begin to memorize the narration the instructor is using. You then use the voice recorder on your phone to re-record the narration. Add words and positive visualization cues that will resonate with you personally. You can then listen to them at your own convenience to build muscle memory when you're off the mats.

Reading and Writing Learners

They prefer learning from written language. When watching tutorials turn the volume all the way down and turn on the closed captioning. You can then read along as the move is being performed. Drawing the moves on paper can also be beneficial. It's not an art contest, so there's no shame if you can't draw well. Reading and writing learners also do well with taking written notes during class and while watching instructional video courses.

Kinesthetic Leaners

They work best with hands on approaches. They often need to 'feel' the technique. If you are watching an instructional you can practice the move simultaneously alongside the video. This can be done solo, with a grappling dummy or live partner (or just simulating it in the air). Try to pay close attention to the body mechanics of the technique. You can also have your partner do the move on you so you can feel all of the nuances of the technique. (Body mechanics, weight distribution, positioning, various points of leverage, etc.)

Kinesthetic leaners will develop muscle memory quickest by executing mindful and purposeful repetitions. Don't just go through the motions, try to feel every aspect of the move. (Both offensively and from a defensive perspective) Hands on learners also perform well when they can engage all of their physical senses. Listening to their partners breathing, feeling and hearing the touch and sound of the gi as they advance in the move can all enhance learning. Because kinesthetic learners "feel" the moves they can adjust quickly to even the subtlest change or discrepancy. This comes in handy when countering or adapting a move on the fly.

Seeing yourself on video also creates a mental image in your brain that you can refer back to later. You can then use that imaging to visualize the technique during mediation or mental rehearsal. The video can be used to identify areas of improvement. During visualization practice you can make those corrections. This will only reinforce the right technique while overriding the former mistakes.

Remember the key with visualization is to immerse yourself in the experience. Use rich, vivid details that ignite all of your senses. What does the technique look like, feel the movements, hear the sounds, get lost in the moment. Remember that the powerful action of visualization triggers the same electrical signals in your brain as if you were actually doing it. Scientists call this "neuromuscular imprinting." You are imbedding the technique into your brain for later translation into the physical world.

One of the greatest values of visualization is you are not encumbered by doing the technique incorrectly. When you physically practice a move you're bound to make mistakes with how you perform it. Many of which will be unconscious initially, but if not addressed can lead to bad habits. With mental imagery you get to completely control the execution of the technique, free from errors. There's obvious benefits to physically doing moves. But if you're alone this can be an excellent alternative or support tool.

In the digital age we now have amazing Jiu-Jitsu content online. In the early days the only option was VHS instructional videos. Now platforms like "BJJ Fanatics" make a world of knowledge accessible from the palm of your hands. Learning from online tutorials offer the advantage of self-paced learning. In a traditional setting you might feel lost in the rhythm of a classroom. But with online learning you can pause, rewind, reflect, take notes, etc. Everything happens at your pace!

Mission:

Use the digital age to supercharge your training, like a tech-savvy training partner who never tires. Discover the magic of video analysis in breaking down your moves, spotting flaws, and polishing your techniques to shine on the mats.

Create a personalized dojo right at home. Whether you're a visual learner mesmerized by the playback, an auditory learner dissecting every detail through commentary, or a kinesthetic learner feeling every move. Set up your space, choose the right gear, and make the most out of every session with the help of your smartphone or camera.

Try the familiarity principle; the more you see and analyze yourself, the more you'll like and refine what you see. It's about building a bridge between old-school grit and new-school tech.

Moderation in Media

Another great benefit with online learning is you get to experience a wider set of teachers, opinions and perspectives. Of course nothing can replace the in-person experience and real-time feedback of a partner or teacher. For many this added supplementation works well for those with busy schedules.

Having access to high level content 24/7 can be very appealing for many enthusiasts. The tricky part with online training is the plethora of instructors, techniques and systems. Even if you isolate your interests to one or two teachers, you still need an effective method of incorporating the material into your BJJ game.

Have you ever gone to a BJJ seminar and after three hours you only remember one technique? This happens to almost everyone.

You've probably heard the famous saying, "**Empty your cup**." It comes from a Zen Buddhism metaphorical lesson called, "The Tea Cup Story." The anecdote illustrates the importance of having an open mind regardless of how much knowledge you've already acquired.

Here's the original version of the story:

A university professor visited Nan-in, a Japanese Zen master, to inquire about Zen. Nan-in served tea. He poured his visitor's cup full, and then kept on pouring. The professor watched the tea overflow until he could no longer restrain himself. "It is overfull. No more will go in!"

"Like this cup," Nan-in said, "**you are full of your own opinions and spec-ulations. How can I show you Zen unless you first empty your cup?**"

In this context the cup represents the mind. The vessel is full of opinions and biases which can impede the ability for growth.

By emptying the cup (clearing it of all preconceived ideas) you are now open to fresh perspectives. This is inherit to all forms of learning. Having a beginner's mind, which suggests a willingness and curiosity to learning, is the key to continuous growth and evolution.

But if we took this a step further and ask, "how do we empty the cup, do we pour out the tea?" You could, but all would then be lost. Instead if you consumed the contents, the cup would naturally become empty.

This passage emphasizes the importance of mindful consumption, partic-ularly in the context of drinking tea. It compares the act of fully experienc-ing and savoring the tea with the less mindful approach where we quickly consume it without appreciation.

The key message is about allowing the body to fully utilize and benefit from the experience, rather than hastily moving on to the next activity or drink without truly relishing in the moment.

The tea, like the lessons we learn in a Jiu-Jitsu classroom, needs time to be introduced and assimilated into our being. A great word for describing this is, automaticity. Another way of saying it would be, autopilot. This is when the doer and the act of doing become one. There's no separation, just complete muscle memory.

But before it can be absorbed, it needs to be tasted.

Taking a moment to enjoy the tea and then ask your body if it's ready for more? When you practice BJJ it's easy to get "information overload." Imagine your brain is like a funnel. If you fill it with too much information, it becomes clogged and nothing can come through. This is why you leave a seminar only remembering one technique. Your funnel is too full.

Mission:

Consume Mindfully. Find balance, knowing when to take in new knowledge, and more importantly, allowing time for that knowledge to simmer and integrate into your repertoire.

Think of each new technique or concept as a sip of tea—savor it, appreciate its nuances, and let it settle before reaching for the next cup.

Micro-Dosing Knowledge

Instead of scrolling social media for 5-10 minutes, educate your curiosities. This expansion of awareness and knowledge grant you access to the next level which means the ability to 'step up' and use the brick in your hand (your phone) to propel you up the success ladder not just on the mats but where it matters most - in life.

Take a move and break it down into four steps. Make it easy enough that you could teach it to a kid in class.

Practice a technique from a certain position or use conceptual learning to build a framework for certain movements.

Curate digital and written notes on your favorite flows .

Watch a video and try the technique or concept yourself .

Dedicate a small time block each day for drilling a specific technique or concept.

Work mobility, flexibility and specific BJJ movements on your own time.

Study etymology. The precision of language. What is it that you're really after? Get to the root of it - go look up the definition of the words you use in Jiu-Jitsu.

Pick up a book and read for five minutes. If that's not your style, listen to a book or watch a video about the summary or review.

Check out new or different ways to engage with the online community of over 40 practitioners through various apps or platforms.

Watch sparring sessions in short segments identifying one area to improve on at a time.

Spar with a specific focus or goal in mind like defending a particular position or going after a certain strangulation.

Ask for immediate, focused feedback on the technique or concept you were just working.

Jot down what did and didn't work each training session.

Spend a few minutes each day mentally rehearsing the general process or exact execution of what you're learning.

Target your conditioning to exercises most utilized in BJJ, such as core strength, flexibility and endurance.

Prioritize recovery, rest, and keep your body in optimal condition for learning and practicing BJJ,

Set specific short-term goals you want to achieve like executing a particular guard pass.

Consider attending a workshop or seminar. These are often more focused and can offer condensed learning opportunities

Take a few minutes and jot down notes in the pages of this book!

Mission:

SHARE three things you've learned through this method and encourage others to do the same. Let's turn our social media into mastery of more than just the scroll.

Survival Expert: RYAN FORD

BJJ Brown Belt and Podcast Host

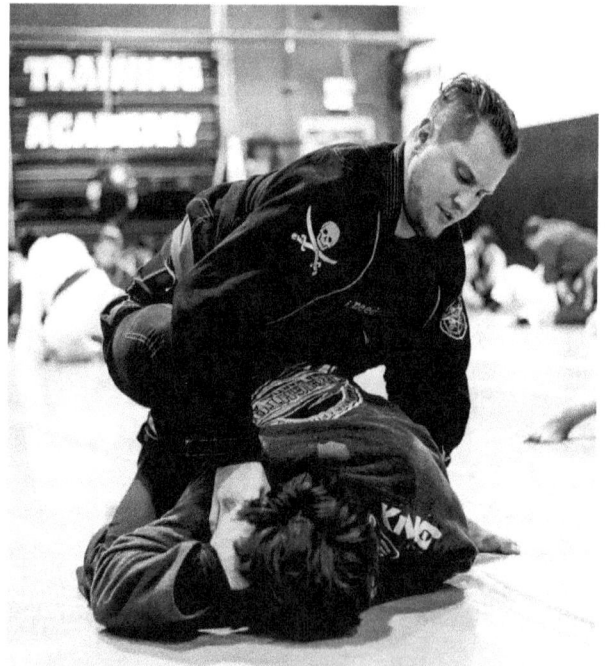

Intel:

The "Grappling Central Podcast" with Ryan Ford was the first BJJ podcast interview that I ever did way back in the day. I was incredibly nervous as his podcast was very popular and one of the first in BJJ. Ryan made me feel more than welcome with his relatable interview style.

Ryan would go on to be the host of the wildly popular BJJ Fanatics podcast. Ryan is an excellent BJJ practitioner with a wealth of experience on the mats. I also respect and honor the amazing insights he's gained by interviewing the best BJJ practitioners and teachers in the world!

Straight from the Source:

My name is Ryan and I am the creator and host of The BJJ Fanatics Podcast, the #1 ranked Brazilian Jiu-Jitsu / Grappling podcast on Apple Podcasts.

In 2015 I launched my show, at the time titled The Grappling Central Podcast, and for 6 years grew it to be the most recognized podcast in the industry.

In 2021, I partnered with industry giant BJJ Fanatics to run the show under their banner and also direct podcasts for their other channels as well, like Fanatic Wrestling, Judo Fanatics and Dynamic Striking.

One of the things that the top guys share is a **focus on improvement**.

They're constantly trying to improve every aspect of their game that they can. They don't sit back on their laurels or past championships. They're always looking for the pieces of the puzzle that are still fuzzy… the pieces that still need sharpening.

The biggest lesson that I've personally taken from any podcast came from Rafael Lovato Jr. He mentioned in passing that he has to *take down notes for everything he ever learns.*

He said he can't comprehend how someone can go into training learn all the details and then go home and just expect to remember it when you've got a family and kids, work life and everything else. That really hit me… I was a purple belt at that time. Ever since then I started keeping a training journal and it completely changed the development of my Jiu-Jitsu. It skyrocketed as a result of taking notes.

A lot of the guys I've interviewed are not former athletes. I assumed early on that I would be talking to guys who played football, wrestled or were at least into physical activities. I'm surprised to see how many non athletic people got into Jiu-Jitsu, and became athletic as a result, and became really good athletes. A lot of these guys are kind of nerdy guys. I mean that in flattering way… they were into comic books, super heroes and stuff like that. They always enjoyed martial arts as something they were interested in. This has changed my perception on the overall landscape of Jiu-Jitsu. When you look at people you think these guys must have been lifelong athletes… but surprisingly most of them have not.

Brazilian Jiu-Jitsu is my life's passion, I have been practicing for fifteen years and have had the privilege to learn from several high level black belts both in the U.S. and in Brazil.

I earned my brown belt from *Professor* Paul Creighton, and despite being sidelined due to the pandemic and balancing raising two kids, I'm currently closing in on earning my black belt.

When I am not working on the podcast, I train avidly in São Paulo, Brazil where I live with my amazing wife and two kids.

I train under UFC legend Demian Maia at his school.

I also enjoy the outdoors, long boarding, music and playing with my son and daughter.

Four Stages of Deep Learning

When we talked about "cognitive load theory" we discussed how our brain only has so much working memory. This is why it's important to limit your viewing time of online BJJ content. We are all inundated with new moves, techniques, etc.

One thing you will notice with my online courses is that I simplify the learning process. I often take what would otherwise be considered complicated sequences and make them easily digestible and accessible. I do this by breaking the techniques down into four simple steps that all build off from one another.

One of the great secrets to teaching is that it's easier to add on to what you already know then to learn something completely new. In BJJ we call this "**chaining techniques**." Instead of bouncing all over the place when I teach, I follow a specific coordinated path. This ensures that I am standing side by side with my audience and not leaving them in the dust.

One of my most influential teaching inspirations is probably not who you'd expect. No it's not Bruce Lee. (Even though I do love him) But this guy didn't practice martial arts at all. It's Bob Ross.

When you watch a Bob Ross painting video he speaks directly to you. Not to an assemblage of beginner or advanced painting enthusiasts. He takes you exactly as you are and speaks in a language that you'll understand. If you've never painted before he invites you to join him step-by-step through the process. If you're more experienced, you're not bored by the depth and subtlety of his techniques. Ross possessed the incredible ability to make complex art principles seem almost intuitive and accessible to everyone. And that's the genius of his approach - he cultivates a learning experience that is inclusive, rewarding, and always progressing. He establishes a connection with his audience and takes them on a journey. He then breaks down the process of painting into easily manageable steps. He talks in a way that is calming and never evokes stress or anxiety. He anticipates the potential challenges while offering solutions along the way. This is analogous to how I approach teaching BJJ. The key word here is accessible. I attempt to take difficult concepts and bring them down to a level of understanding that's attainable for all. But how is this accomplished?

I've created a template for rapidly integrating complex moves into your game.

I call it the "**Four stages of deep learning**":

1. **Demonstration**

2. **Deconstruction**

3. **Comprehension**

4. **Performance**

To understand the move is to assimilate it. With it becomes a deep connection between intellectual understanding and embodied practice. It's not just about parroting the move robotically. True comprehension means a deep acknowledgment of its underlying principles, variations and subtleties.

If you were in a classroom I would first demonstrate the technique so you have some context to refer back to. During this stage we will identify and memorize the four steps of the move. If your teacher doesn't teach in four steps, try to isolate them as they speak.

Stage One: Demonstration

During stage one you would be drilling with your partner. If you're alone you can be viewing the video over and over, but with the volume turned down. The objective is to focus exclusively on the 'how' and 'why' of the movements. If you are practicing with a live partner (or grappling dummy) verbally state each step as you perform them. For example: if it's an armbar from the mount you would say, "1. Secure the arm, 2. Opposite leg posted, 3. Leg over the head, 4. Control the joint and elevate the hips." If you're in a classroom you can silently speak your four steps under your breath.

While practicing from stage one it would be worthwhile, whenever possible, to video record the execution of the technique. Don't record the first set of repetitions. Try to get into a good flow and then record yourself. If you're at home with a grappling dummy, it's an even better opportunity because nobody else is watching.

Stage Two: Deconstruction

You'll now want to review your recording. As you assess your technique you should break it into three criteria: P.C.M. Prepare, Condense, Modify. During the preparation portion you are identifying the four steps to the technique. Does each movement look clean, effortless and smooth. Or can you find flaws in your movements.

Now condense those flaws into even smaller pieces. This will allow you to focus on each error individually rather than getting overwhelmed by the entire technique. Each flaw is now a singular problem to be solved, rather than a part of a larger, more complex issue.

You can do drills that isolate and target areas that need attention. For example: You might find that during the execution of the technique your foot might be slightly off which is rendering the move ineffective. So you then rework the technique to account for this adjustment.

The final step is to modify. Now you can make adjustments in the technique that fit your body better. This could be an adjustment of a grip or how your place a limb, etc. The goal isn't to make huge, sweeping changes all at once. It's about small incremental improvements that lead to an effortless execution of the move.

Once you have drilled the adjustments you've made, then you'll need to re-film the technique. The great thing about video his that it is a clear, objective representation of the move. There's no relying on memory, feelings or room for subjective evaluations. There's just you performing it plain and simple. The beauty is that you can rewind and pause as many times you need to.

When you review your second version of the move you'll want to look at even more details. The objective is to get the technique as close a rendition as possible to the source material. You don't have to reach perfection, but you certainly can strive for it.

Stage Three: Comprehension

As a result of the drilling that happens in stage two, it prepares you for stage three which is comprehension. But to truly 'understand' something the perfect litmus test is to teach it to another person. When you share something new with another student it forces you to go deeper into the move. You must now understand every detail, anticipate common questions or problems, and explain it in a clear, effective manner. Being able to articulate something requires a deep, comprehensive understanding of the material. Teaching also forces you to see gaps in your own technique that may need addressing. There's a great saying, "To teach is to learn twice." Or as I continually preach, "Teaching is learning on steroids!"

If you don't have a physical partner to teach, then you can write out the steps as if your were sharing it with another. Document each step of the technique along with a narrative on how you would teach it.

For example:

Version 1.0:

Technique - armbar from the mount

Control the arm - Demonstrate that you need to initially control the shoulder and elbow.

Post the opposite leg - Show them that as you post the opposite leg you have to rotate your hips 180 degrees (semi circle).

Leg over the head - As the leg goes over the head you want to keep your hips hovering slightly above their body narrowly making contact.

Lay back and elevate your hips - As you finish the armbar you want to control all three joints. The wrist, elbow and shoulder.

This exercise should be repeated multiples times to isolate the details of the technique. For example you may have 4-5 versions each with features that build upon the previous iterations.

Version 2.0:

Control the arm - As you reach under the shoulder you'll want to lift it from the floor. As you elevate the joint, slide your same side knee into the space you've created.

Post the opposite leg - As you slide your knee around, place it under their head like a pillow. Your opposite side knee will be posted and tight to their body.

Leg over the head - Before you slide the leg over the head be sure to post your same side hand on their head. Make sure that your leg clears their head before your butt hits the ground. Lay back and elevate your hips - Squeeze your knees and adductor muscles (inside your thighs). This will lock their joint into place and amplify the pressure.

As you can see I have added additional relevant details that are ultimately crucial to overall makeup of the technique. Regardless of their importance, we still need to introduce them in layers. If we dumped all of those important attributes into the move at version 1.0 we would experience information overload. The human brain is an amazing piece of technology, but can only handle so much new information all at once.

Scientists believe that the working memory of a person, which is used to process and manipulate knowledge, has a limited amount of space. They have calculated that the human brain can hold about seven pieces of new information (plus or minus two). A normal phone number is ten digits. Some people may find it challenging to individually memorize ten numbers. But if they employed techniques like "chunking" the numbers together, or using rhyme, they may improve the results.

It's important to note that this isn't always directly translatable to learning larger quantities of information over time, like Jiu-Jitsu. Learning information that is a part of a larger framework can expedite the process. Think of each technique as piece of a puzzle that makes up a much larger image. Always be on the lookout for where each new technique you're learning fits into your overall game (framework).

Stage Four: Performance

There are two levels to performance.

1. You want to be able to properly demonstrate the technique on an uke (non-resisting partner).

2. Be able to problem solve and test the technique under hostile and semi-hostile conditions.

Once you can perform the technique, hitting all the key points, you'll want to pressure test it. You can do this under semi-controlled conditions where your partner purposely creates roadblocks and obstacles. If you're drilling the armbar from the mount you could start from side control. Your objective would be to transition to the mount and execute an armbar. Your partners job is to offer varying levels of resistance. You can decide ahead of time how much opposition will be given.

For example you could both agree that you'll move at 30 - 40% speed and resistance. This allows for a more dedicated learning experience. If you start at 100%, it will be challenging to engage in any opportunities for expansion.

Another viable option is to find partners during open mat to test your techniques on. If they are better than you or at an equal level, it will be hard to do this effectively. You'll want to find someone that can offer you a decent competitive roll, but ultimately you can control the outcome. For upper levels, brown and black belts - purple and blue belts are perfect to practice on during live rolls. White belts may be too unrefined to offer the right challenges.

Purple belts may find that blue belts are perfect for live drilling. Blue belts may find that white belts with 3-4 stripes are suitable. White belts can work with lower level beginners (1-2 stripes), but not absolute novices. It can be dangerous to "test out" moves that you're still learning on newbies. If you are a novice, drill your new moves on uke's (drilling partners), not during live rolling.

If you're a beginner, always leave room for your partner to either escape or tap out. When you're just getting started, it's best to 'catch and release' the move until you have mastered the subtleties of the technique.

As you begin to implement your new technique into your game, you'll want to address every possible 'what if' scenario. If you don't know the list of possibilities, don't worry. You will discover them when you are pressure testing the move during live rolling. As you test your move on varying partners, you'll discover new roadblocks and opportunities.

Remember, learning a technique doesn't have an ending point. You will constantly be refining, updating and adding to your technique. Think of it like getting an "update" on your phone. I believe that Jiu-Jitsu moves are living, breathing entities. You have to constantly look at them, play with them, dust them off, sharpen them, etc, Like a seed that was once planted. Even though it may have grown bigger, it still needs water.

Mission:

For practice it would be ideal to have a home BJJ training area. We all have different living situations so for some this may not be realistic. You can however modify and make it work! The most important thing isn't really having mats, but rather a half way decent grappling dummy. You can find something that will work for under $100 on Amazon. If you have hard floors it would be worth it to purchase a small folding mat or some puzzle mats. Even carpeted floor will be sufficient. This doesn't have to be a substantial investment, you just need a little space to drill.

One of the most significant ways to accelerate improvement is to video record yourself practicing and drilling with partners. This method can offer crucial insights into your training. When we rely solely on memories of previous experiences, our perceptions can be distorted by biases. However, reviewing footage provides a third-person perspective, enabling a more objective viewpoint. You see things as they really are, not how you perceived them during the roll. As you view and study your rolling and drilling you'll want to utilize the tips we provided on learning styles.

We embody a mix of different learning styles, and we have the ability to enhance those in which we are less proficient. By investigating various learning preferences, you can craft the perfect learning environment, irrespective of how others present the material. I have personally experienced BJJ environments where the teaching style didn't align with my learning preferences. As someone who thrives on a combination of kinesthetic and visual learning, I find that excessive verbal explanations can be disengaging. I have taught myself to block out the "noise" and focus completely on visually absorbing the move. For this mission, start by delving deeper into understanding your preferred learning styles. Discover the ideal blend that truly resonates with you. Then, begin to explore other learning modalities to broaden your horizons and enhance your overall learning capacity. Apply these into your classroom experience along with your home drilling.

Begin applying the "four stages of deep learning" into your in-class and at-home practice sessions. This approach will accelerate your learning process and help develop your muscle memory. Ensure you have a home grappling dummy and set up a training area at home. It can be as simple as storing the dummy behind the couch after your drill sessions. Video record yourself practicing the techniques you're currently focusing on. If feasible, record your grappling sessions in class as well. You can review the footage alone, with your partner, or with your instructor during a private lesson. Each of these methods will yield valuable insights. Utilize all of our suggestions for reviewing and internalizing the material!

The Evolution of Modern BJJ

Gone are the days when the same old techniques were all you needed. Today, the art is vibrant and constantly evolving with fresh moves and strategies. Let's step onto 'the Mat of Continuous Learning' together:

Stay curious. The world of BJJ doesn't stand still, and neither should you. Immerse yourself in the latest matches, find fellow practitioners who are redefining the game and platforms that showcase cutting-edge techniques.

Identify new guards, passes, and submissions that resonate with the modern competitor's playbook. Incorporate these into your training one move at a time. Whether it's mastering the intricacies of the worm guard or unraveling the complexities of modern leg entanglements, take it slow and ensure each new technique is done with understanding and precision.

Bring these new techniques into the open mat. This is your canvas, where you paint your movements against various partners. Pay attention to the details, the reactions, and the effectiveness of each move. Adjust, adapt, and refine.

BJJ often demands a unique set of physical qualities. Whether it's the flexibility required to maneuver through guards or the explosive power for passes, tailor your conditioning to support your technical growth. Integrating yoga or pilates can enhance your flexibility, while a kettlebell routine might build the core strength necessary for those power moves.

After each session, take a moment to reflect. Review your sparring videos, jot down insights in your journal, and discuss them with your coach or training partners. This reflection is your whetstone, sharpening your skills and honing your understanding.

Keep your mental agility as keen as your physical skills. Modern BJJ requires not just physical adaptation but also cognitive flexibility. Embrace the mindset that every challenge is an opportunity to learn and grow.

As you acquire new knowledge, share it with your tribe. Teaching is not just an act of giving but a process of reinforcing your own learning. Start a study group, lead a seminar, and help others in your age group navigate the evolving landscape of BJJ.

Regularly reevaluate your goals and the effectiveness of your training strategies. Are the new techniques serving you well? Are there adjustments to be made? This continual reassessment ensures that your BJJ journey is not just about keeping pace but setting the pace.

Have fun staying engaged with modern trends. Be bold in bringing new vigor and wisdom to every roll. Let's keep rolling, adapting, and evolving, because in Jiu-Jitsu, as in life, the only constant is change. Welcome to the evolution, warriors!

Mission:

Experimentation on the mat is crucial; use open mat sessions as a canvas to test and refine these techniques, ensuring they resonate with modern standards.

Strengthen your physical foundation with targeted exercises like yoga for flexibility and kettlebells for core strength, supporting your technical growth and preparing you for rigorous rolls.

Reflect on your practice through video analysis and note-taking, discussing insights with coaches or peers to sharpen your understanding and execution of techniques.

Maintain cognitive flexibility to adapt to new challenges and share your knowledge to reinforce learning and assist others.

Regular reassessment of your training strategies and goals ensures you not only keep pace with BJJ's evolution but also lead in its development. It is a continuous cycle of learning, testing, and refining to thrive in the modern landscape of Brazilian Jiu-Jitsu.

Debriefing Assessment:

Evaluate how technology has influenced your BJJ learning and training regimen. Reflect on your media consumption and its impact on your training focus and knowledge acquisition.

The focus is on personal growth, adaptability, and the continuous pursuit of mastery in the art of Jiu-Jitsu.

The journey into tech-enhanced BJJ training has revolutionized our approach to learning. Tools like video analysis software, mobile apps for technique drills, and online seminars have allowed us to customize our training environment. Reflecting on these tools, assess how they have specifically influenced your practice routines and your ability to integrate new techniques into your repertoire.

In the age of information overload, finding balance in our media consumption is crucial. This chapter encourages a reflection on how the media we consume impacts our focus and mental clarity during training. Consider how selective engagement with content—choosing quality over quantity—has affected your mental readiness and overall training effectiveness.

Adopting the concept of micro-dosing knowledge, where learning is broken down into small, manageable segments, can lead to more sustainable and long-term retention of techniques. Evaluate how incorporating short, focused snippets of learning (via apps, podcasts, or quick video tutorials) has enhanced your understanding and execution of complex BJJ maneuvers.

The deep learning process in BJJ can be transformative, especially when facilitated by digital platforms. From initial exposure to concepts to achieving mastery, digital tools enable a layered learning experience. Reflect on the stages you've navigated—Unconscious Incompetence, Conscious Incompetence, Conscious Competence, and Unconscious Competence—and how technology has supported your progression in each stage.

PART II:
ON THE MATS -
STRATEGIES FOR PHYSICAL
ENGAGEMENT

Operations:
Field Work

Practical advice for daily training, hygiene, dealing with injuries, and understanding the social dynamics of BJJ gyms.

Scan the QR code for real-world applications and field training exercises.
https://www.youtube.com/playlist?list=PLwb5iQup9938sngm-hJwF-NzCpf-W1Qsbw

Belts, Stripes and Progression

First we must dispel the most annoying myth in the martial arts regarding the origin of the colored belts. You may have heard this little tale, or some version of it?

In the old days, everyone started with a white belt and as time progressed the belt got dirty from use. First with green grass stains, then brown from the dirt and eventually black from years of use. Then as time went on the black color wore away revealing white underneath, signifying the return of the master to his roots. Fun story, but not true.

The grading system used today in modern BJJ schools has its origins from the martial art of Judo. The belt system in Judo was created by its founder Jigoro Kano in the late 19th century. Initially there were only white and black belts awarded and no colored belts. White represented a beginner, whereas black was a more advanced student.

Kawaishi, who brought Judo to Europe in the 1920s. He found that western students needed a visual representation to understand advancement and as a motivation. This innovation was widely adopted in other martial arts at the time.

Initially Brazilian Jiu-Jitsu only had four colored belts. White, light blue (instructors), black belt, dark blue (masters). The modern BJJ belt system was formalized by the International Brazilian Jiu-Jitsu Federation (I.B.J.J.F.) in the early 2000's, and then widely adopted by the worldwide

BJJ community.

Grading in Brazilian Jiu-Jitsu isn't as formalized as other martial arts. The process of awarding belts can differ greatly from teacher to teacher. Some schools test on very specific curriculum where others do a more "spur of the moment", time-based method. Both are valuable in different ways. Some people like the more formal version where you meet and test on blocks of curriculum. Others may find the spontaneous approach more representative of the ever-changing nature of Brazilian Jiu-Jitsu.

In an organized grading system, each belt level has a clear set of skills to learn. A student knows exactly what they need to acquire to move on to the next level. This is helpful because it makes things clear and lets you focus on specific techniques or skillsets. This method can be especially helpful for beginners, who may learn best when they have a plan for 'how to learn.' It gives them a clear set of goals and skills to work toward, which can be encouraging and help guide their training.

Conversely a more spontaneous approach has its own benefits. In this model, the teacher might decide to promote a student based on how well they do in class and sparring sessions as a whole instead of how well they know a certain set of skills. This method may not follow a clear set of standards, but it does correlate directly to someones performance during live grappling. Which is arguably the 'best' metric at the end of the day.

A school that follows a more self-defense focused approach to BJJ will likely follow a more organized curriculum. Whereas tournament oriented schools tend to follow a more spur of the moment approach to belt promotions. Sometimes you may even see belts get awarded on the podium at tournaments based on someones performance. Regardless of how belts are presented, just about every professor shares the same goal to improve their students life through this amazing martial art.

Another tradition followed by some schools is the gauntlet. Also known as the "shark tank" or the "belt whipping" ceremony. The ritual is that when someone is newly promoted they walk, shirtless through a line of team-mates who strike them with their belts. Sometimes participants will hit lightly and other times they will swing for the fences and leave a mark.

The origins of the gauntlet are a bit murky and cannot be substantiated. It has the likeness to military traditions of hazing individuals to mark a milestone and foster camaraderie. Some in the BJJ community believe strongly that it's an outdated, unnecessary tradition. While others may feel it's harmless. Regardless, it should always be up to the individual if they want to participate.

The time you spend at each belt level can vary widely from person to person. This is why your professor will probably tell you, "don't ever compare your progress to others as it's such an individual journey." The I.B.J.J.F. offers guidelines for how much time should be spent at each belt level. But ultimately it really comes down to the individual student and professor.

Adult belt colors in Brazilian Jiu-Jitsu:

White - Blue - Purple - Brown - Black - Coral - Red

Stripes and the Green belt -

Stripes or tips represent small incremental steps in your progress. Most academies use four stripes on each belt. Stripes are typically a piece of white tape wrapped around the stripe bar. If the tape falls off just ask your professor to perform the "re-striping" ceremony at your next visit. (No I'm just kidding, just put a new piece on yourself)

Some schools use a green belt at the white belt level in lieu of the fourth stripe. (Normally the green belt is used as an official belt for teens aged 14 and older)

White belt -

"The baby years" They don't know what they don't know. The beginning level of most martial arts systems. Often representing innocence and taking your first baby steps in BJJ. This is a time where basic moves are understood and refined. This is literally the building of the foundation upon which the proverbial house will stand (or fall). With the white belt comes a sense of humility for this deep, complex art.

Blue belt -

"The toddler years" After learning the fundamental concepts that underscore BJJ, you are now mastering how to walk, run and jump. Like a child you may fall from time to time, but you are now learning from your mistakes. You are beginning to experiment with different concepts and ideas. With this level comes accomplishment, but also frustration as upper belts (adults in the case of our metaphor) now treat you differently. There's an expectation that comes with blue belt. Both from the wearer and those you train with and under.

Purple belt -

"The teen years" Like a teenager, you are beginning to develop your identity and perception of who you'll become. You are maturing and creating your own game. You may take greater risks with even more profound results. But like a teenager, you have all the freedom and responsibility of an adult but without the life experience. Even though you're no longer bound by your teacher (the "adults" around you) you still need them to progress.

Brown belt -

"Growing up" This is the stage of maturity where you are preparing your-self for the "real world" of adulthood. In preparation for black belt you're now polishing and perfecting your technique. You understand the details and subtleties that make a significant difference in the execution and success of moves. It's no longer about the collection of new techniques at this level, but developing mastery with what you already know. You now understand the art on a deeper level and can share it with others.

Black Belt -

"Adulthood" With this stage comes the role of sharing the art with others. As a budding professor and teacher of BJJ there comes great power and even greater responsibility. A good teacher can share the art with anyone regardless of skill or physical capabilities, making it accessible to all. As a black belt you are not only expected to be physically competent, but to embody the core concepts of BJJ: perseverance, respect and discipline. In the "adulthood" phase you further recognize the importance of always being a student and continuing to challenge yourself. Remember, as a black belt you're now the guardian of the tradition, culture and history of Jiu-Jitsu.

Beyond black…"Ambassador of the Art" I'm am a decade into being a BJJ black belt. I don't know what is beyond black. But I will say this, I have learned more in my time as a BJJ black belt than I did all the time I spent at brown.

My belt story. I started my BJJ journey in 1996. But I had already been grappling for a few years. I was previously a black belt in other traditional martial arts and would often meet friends and train. But in the Summer of 1996 I took an M.M.A. fight (then known as N.H.B. or No Holds Barred Fighting). I lost the match to a blue belt in BJJ. It was an eye opener for me and was the official beginning of my Jiu-Jitsu journey.

I started as a white belt, but was promoted to purple in 1999 by my then BJJ professor Allan Goes. So no, I was never a blue belt. It wasn't that I was a super star student either. But training back then was very different. All we did was train BJJ day and night. I would go onto receive my brown belt in 2001, and then my black belt in 2014.

Whenever someone hears this story they will immediately respond with, "Why were you a brown belt so long? and were you training the entire time?" The answer is yes and yes. I started at lightening speed and then slowed to a snails pace. My challenge was a combination of factors. I had moved with my family a few times. When you start somewhere new again you have to build a relationship with the instructor. Trust and rapport are not built in a day. Different instructors have different expectations and teaching methodologies. Every time you start somewhere new, you start all over again. Each academy has different curriculum, focus and teaching styles.

I was also going through bouts of depression which often got in the way of my Jiu-Jitsu training. Depression would often cast a long, dark shadow over my training. It would sap my energy and motivation. My breakthrough finally came when I used the lessons on the mat to help me navigate my emotional challenges. I viewed depression like any BJJ opponent. It was often cunning, unpredictable and would constantly test my mental and physical strength. I knew it had the ability to put me in uncomfortable positions and blur my focus. Just like in BJJ where you study and predict your adversary's next move. I began to understand my own battle with depression.

I approached it from a strategic BJJ perspective. The first lesson in BJJ is to never show your back. I understood, for the first time that opponents must be faced head on. Where each BJJ match is a learning opportunity to study your partners habits and tendencies. I began to recognize my own depression triggers. Like BJJ training, dealing with depression is a long-game. It's something that can be managed on an ongoing basis, but like a tough opponent, it should never be underestimated. Armed with a new perspective I saw my depression episodes not as set-backs, but as opportunities for growth and expansion.

By making changes in my life like: improving my diet, better sleep, getting consistent and regular training, starting a mindfulness meditation practice have all helped me with this challenge. My long tenure at brown belt wasn't so much about the time at the belt, but about eventually utilizing the tools and skills I had developed on the mat to face this formidable opponent. When I reflect on my own journey I am grateful for every drop of blood, sweat and tears. The lesson isn't to NOT care about the belts. As much as it isn't to only care about the belts. You have to strike the right balance for your life. The belts are important milestones that can be helpful in guiding you to your goals. They represent the fruits of your hard work, commitment and resilience. It's important to celebrate your victories, but to continue to seek a growth mind-set. Embrace the struggle and expansion that comes with it. I will tell you that as a black belt it doesn't get any easier. You just get better.

What to do if you're stuck at a belt. Create a dialogue with your instructor to understand your best path to progression. It's important to communicate your questions clearly to your coaches. A good place to start from would be, "What can I be doing to progress in my training?" Remember, they are there to support and guide you. It would be worthwhile to schedule a private lesson with your teacher to discuss strategies for your success.

Don't rely on feedback from your instructor alone. Seek the opinions of your training partners. They probably know you better than anyone and can offer valuable insights into your strengths and weaknesses. You can expand on this by trying collaborative or mutual learning. This is a modality where you roll with your partners and then immediately discuss what happened and offer each other advice. This is a great way to get deeper understanding into your training while building camaraderie with your teammates.

Regardless of where you're today in your BJJ journey, don't give up. I was a brown belt for thirteen years. I know the frustration that comes with belts. It's not a race to the finish. Enjoy and embrace the path you're on. It's not about the stripes or belts, it's the accumulation and mastery of knowledge. Focus on that and everything will fall into place.

A simple, but realistic belt progression outline for BJJ:

White belt to blue belt, 1.5 - 2 years

Blue - purple, 3-4 years

Purple - brown, 3-4 years

Brown - black, 3-4 years

Mission:

In BJJ, you cannot escape the importance of belts, as progressing through them is essential to excelling in this art. It's similar to attending college but saying, "no thanks" to the degree that accompanies it. The problem with the college scenario is that the school wouldn't let you learn the next set of material without first proving yourself by passing your courses. You wouldn't be allowed to move forward without first completing the previous material. First you get an associates degree, then bachelors, then a masters and eventually a p.h.D. This can take 10-13 years of total schooling. This is very much like the BJJ journey which can also take 10-15 years. The difference in academics is that everyone follows the same exact path. BJJ is far more subjective and based on a different set of metrics. But there are similarities that are worth noting. You cannot escape the belts nor the progression and personal evolution that accompanies them.

Document in your BJJ notebook your short-term and long-term goals related to your belt progression. Short term - List the specific steps that can be taken to help you improve your BJJ practice in the next 3-6 months. Action steps: taking notes, writing out the steps of moves, video analysis of competition / grappling or move execution, scheduling a private lesson and setting goals with your professor, etc. Long term - Where do you see your progression in the next 1, 2 and 5 years down the road? This could be tournaments, new belt levels, developing certain aspects of your game, teaching and coaching, opening a school, etc.

The I in Team:
Cleanliness and Hygiene

The importance of good hygiene and BJJ cannot be understated. Grappling is a stinky, messy martial art. You're constantly exchanging sweat and body fluids with a group of other adults and teens. You'll get dripped on and repeatedly sloshed in a sea of sweat. The funny thing is that BJJ is such an addiction, that we somehow become "okay" with it. But don't get too comfortable as skin infections can be serious business.

The Top Four skin infections from Grappling sports:

Ring Worm -

'Tinea corporis' is a fungal infection that appears as a red, itchy rash that forms a distinct circle with a clear center. This is probably the most common skin infection grapplers experience. Never roll with someone who has ringworm (or hiding it behind a suspicious bandage).

Prevention - Wash and scrub exposed skin before and after class with antibacterial soap. Keep nails neatly trimmed. Always shower immediately and wash all training gear, uniforms, joint sleeves after class. Don't let your gi sit over night to dry with with sweat on it. Never share towels or training gear with teammates. Many BJJ students swear by using "Head and Shoulders" shampoo as a hair and body wash after training as a preventative measure. The most important preventative measure you can take is to clean thoroughly after class!

Impetigo is a skin infection caused by Staphylococcus or Streptococcus bacteria that spreads easily from person to person. It manifests as red sores or blisters that break open, ooze, and eventually crust over in a yellowish brown color.

Prevention - Maintain good personal hygiene and shower with antibacterial soap before and after training. Clean and cover any cuts, scrapes, or abrasions promptly. Wash and disinfect training gear and equipment after each use. Avoid skin-to-skin contact with anyone showing signs of impetigo. If you suspect you have impetigo, seek medical treatment and avoid training until it has cleared.

Staph infection (Staphylococcus aureus) -

The red, inflamed pimples or boils that result from a Staphylococcus infection can be very painful. Staph infections can develop into life-threatening crises if not treated promptly. Contact a health care professional immediately, never wait.

Prevention - Wash and clean with antibacterial soap before and after training. Maintain a healthy barrier by washing and moisturizing your skin regularly. *Never pick or scratch pimples, sores or ingrown hairs on your skin* Never train with someone you suspect may be covering something up.

Herpes Gladiatorum "Mat Herpes" - This is an HSV-1 skin infection that manifests as painful blisters or sores filled with fluid. It spreads easily from person to person and can also be picked up from contaminated surfaces.

Prevention - Like the previously mentioned skin infections, always keep yourself and your gear clean. Shower immediately after training. Never go home, wait and then shower. (Or worse, go to bed and don't shower) If you don't have access to a shower at your academy, at least wash all of your exposed skin before you leave and change into dry, clean clothing.

Maintaining hygiene in the gym isn't just courtesy; it's crucial for health and performance. Here's how to be a hero of cleanliness:

Gear Up Right: Always use freshly washed gear and uniforms.

Mat Manners: Wipe down mats before and after use with disinfectant – your training partners will thank you.

Personal Cleanse: A quick pre-training shower minimizes the spread of bacteria and post-training shower is a must to ward off infections.

Keeping your gear clean and sanitized!

Don't wait! Wash your gear as soon as you get home. Don't dump your wet gi into a basket and leave it. Or worse, leave it in your car to dry. This is a recipe for a skin infection, plus you'll have more trouble getting the stink from your gi later. If it's extra smelly, add a cup or white vinegar to the wash for added defense. You can even leave your gear in the wash to soak over night. Throw everything in the wash. Rash guards, spats, gi, belt and flip flops.

When your gear comes out of the wash shake it out aggressively. This will get out any wrinkles and gets it back to it's original shape. If you're tall like me you can stand on the pant leg and stretch them out while they're still wet. You can do the same with the top as well. It's helps it stretch back out to its former glory. If you're a tall practitioner be warned, most gi's shrink in the dryer. R.I.P. - I have lost many a good BJJ uniform to the dryer!

Protective gear such as mouth guards and knee pads (this includes ankle, elbow and knee sleeves) should be cleaned and sanitized on a regular basis. Use a dental sanitizer or a solution of water and mouthwash to clean your mouthpiece. After each usage, spray or wipe clean the protective gear with a disinfectant and let it air dry. This leads to the next question. "Should you wear a mouthpiece when grappling?" The answer is simple: A mouth piece is cheaper than dental work. (Less painful too)

One of the most "controversial" topics in BJJ leaves me the most befuddled. What's the question? "Should I wash my coveted BJJ belt?" Some will say, "Absolutely not, you'll wash away the knowledge!" Others, will quickly respond with, "**Hogwash!** It's a piece of cloth!" But the facts are the facts. **Your belt, like your gi and rash guard, will become a breeding ground for bacteria if left uncleaned**. Over time the build up of dirt, sweat and skin will develop some funky odors. To minimize the smell you can hang your belt from a coat hanger and spray it with disinfectant. Washing can be done by hand with a gentle detergent or in the washing machine using a garment bag. *If all of your knowledge disappears down the drain then we apologize in advance. (Remember, bad smells indicate the presence of bacteria)

It's important that *ALL* of your gear get the class-A cleaning treatment. This includes your gym bag which can be the worst offender. A mesh bag is an excellent alternative for a sweaty, wet gi and towel. Speaking of towel, if you're a sweater like me, always have a hand towel nearby when you're training. Although some may be reluctant to wash their belts due to superstitious reasons. Doing so is essential for preventing skin infections and being respectful of those you share the mat with.

If you feel like you've tried everything and your gi still smells:

'How to' strip wash a gi / rash guard / spats that smells horrific!

Step 1: Pre-Soak - Fill a big container (like a bathtub) with warm water and add white vinegar until the gi is completely submerged. If you want the best effect, soak your uniform / rash guards in the vinegar solution for at least two to four hours and preferably overnight. Vinegar eliminates odor by killing the germs that produce it.

Step 2: After the pre-soak, remove the gi from the vinegar solution and put it into the washing machine with detergent and one half cup of baking soda. (This will act as a natural deodorizer that can help remove any unpleasant odors) Warm or cool water is best as hot water can shrink the fabric or even destroy it. Wash on a gentle cycle.

Step 3: Use an enzymatic sports laundry detergent made specifically to eliminate perspiration bacteria smells. These detergents have enzymes that specifically attack odor molecules and degrade them.

Step 4: After the gi is washed, try to dry it in natural sunlight. The sunlight can help further eliminate bacteria. Plus it will smell fresh!

Step 5: Once the gi is dry, inspect it for any remaining stench. If it still smells, try rewashing it a second time. If the smell still lingers, immediately bury it in your back yard!

<u>Top Cleanliness Quick Tips!</u>

- Always carry mints and mouth wash in your bag.
- Wash your hands regularly, especially after restroom visits. Always wear flip flops in bathrooms and disinfect the bottom of your feet before returning to the training mats. (Keep a small container of hand sanitizer attached to your gym bag)
- Trim finger and toe nails regularly.

- Keep your ears clean and free from wax buildup.

- Put on fresh deodorant before class. (Maybe even spread that deodorizer around your private areas too)

- Wear a rash guard under your gi. Nobody likes sweaty, wet chest hair in their face. If you're not hairy, nobody likes to "slip and slide" off your bare chest either! (If you sweat, bring a clean hand towel)

- Practice good foot hygiene. Toe nails trimmed. Keep your feet covered if you have any foot conditions like athletes foot. (Treat immediately & never share nail clippers)

- Disinfect and wash all of your gear after each session. (Gi's, rash guards, spats / tights, gym bag, joint sleeves, etc.)

- Stay home if you're sick. Nobody wants you to "sweat out your cold" on them. And don't try to convince anyone those are allergies!

- Never train with skin infections. Check your own skin regularly.

Mission:

Wash everything, including your belt. Your's and your partners skin health and personal hygiene is the ultimate priority.

Survival Expert: MARCO LALA

Number of years active: 43, Instructors/ pedigree:
Karate, Grand Master Shigeru Oyama / Master Kiohi-
ko Hioki Judo, Shiro Oishi BJJ, Master Edson Carvalho (Carlson Gracie / Mehdi and Carvalho Sr.)

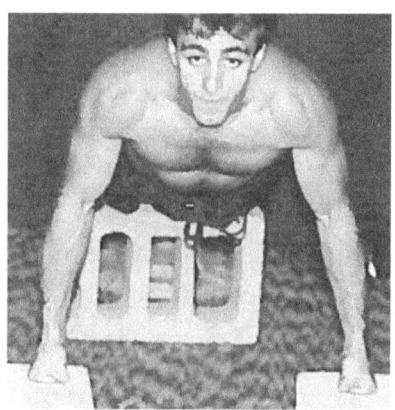

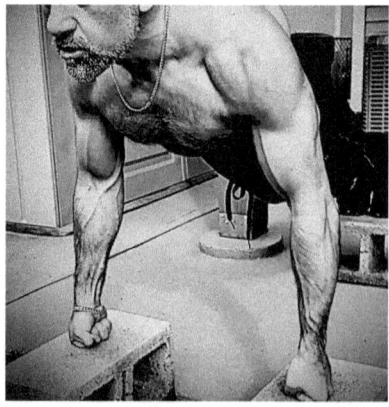

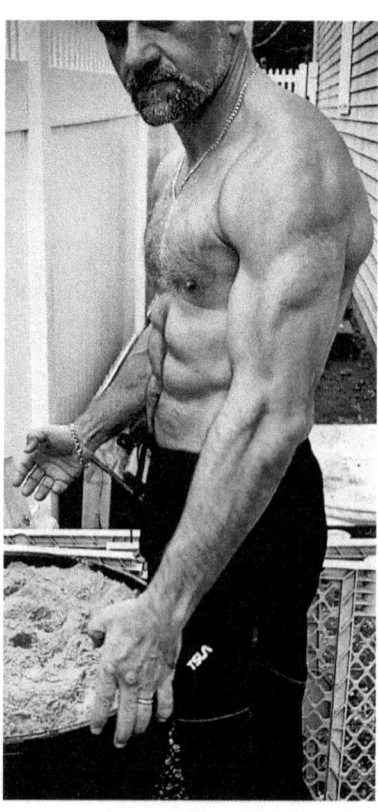

Intel:

A longtime martial artist and respected figure in the BJJ community that is now in his mid 50's but looks like a much younger athlete. He's one of the first martial artists in the United States to offer instructional video courses way back in the early days. I fondly remember seeing his ad's in black belt magazine in the early 1990's on achieving the splits and knocking his opponents out in seconds!

He earned a black belt certification at the young age of 17 in Kyokushin Karate (the strongest and toughest Karate system in the world). By the time he was 18 he had written three books on martial arts. Marco became one of the youngest "non-Asian," Bare Knuckle Full Contact champions at only 21 in 1987 (recorded live on the „Knock Out Any Attacker" video series). Marco is also a black belt in Judo and Brazilian Jiu-Jitsu. He is also the founder of his own system, Tettsu Bushi Jitsu.

Marco is currently one of the most active investment property specialists in the New York area. He has personally handled the sale of over 1.7 billion in the New York Metropolitan area.

From the Source:

Cross training for over 40 athletes is absolutely critical to excel in the martial arts. The fusion of strength, flexibility, mobility, explosiveness, endurance have to be forged through all means of physical training. Proper weight training is underrated in the martial arts as it was always associated with bodybuilding. It's critical for every physical endeavor and a better quality of life as one ages if done properly.

Although mostly "unintentional" there were brief periods of my life where I pursued building a dojo and also a bachelors degree and ultimately a professional career in commercial real estate where I may have also been fortunate enough to prevent extensive joint, neck and physical damage with overtraining and high contact fighting.

I think I've learned to balance myself as I got older as extreme training and physical tests were always a part of our training. Especially more so with the Karate breaking techniques and body conditioning. I feel lucky that I did Judo religiously before BJJ as the falls, throws and ukemi are more damaging to the body. It was a great foundation for training with a Judo based BJJ instructor as Edson Carvalho. I think his Carlson based approach to balanced randori / newaza was critical.

I stay healthy by controlling food portions and also stick to a strict bicycling and stretching routine. I also religiously see my physician and get regular blood work. I have never tried nor will do PEDS, I limit my alcohol consumption, and stay away from all recreational drugs.

An unexpected benefit I've discovered is how using my mind and strategy to nullify attacks from more aggressive training partners allows me to keep thinking on my feet outside the dojo. *Whether in the office, board room or on a sales call, I'm always applying Jiu-Jitsu in a way in all my dealings.*

The thing that inspires me most about training over 40, now over 55... and beyond is the how the *daily stresses seem to melt away on the mat,* and the challenge to make my technique less reliant of pure physical attributes although it's a challenge with the young guns. I just have fun and like getting into bad positions to work escapes and surviving. Sometime you can even catch 'em!

Stress in Jiu-Jitsu

We can't go into stress, on or off the mats, without putting our focus on breath control and awareness techniques. There's nothing more important than breathing (literally). Not only is it important for your survival, but it can be used as a tool to enhance your performance. Let's first discuss when to breathe 'In' and when to breathe 'Out.' A simple, but powerful rule is to always inhale when your head is moving away from your feet. Your exhalation (out breath) should always coincide with your head moving towards your feet.

From a more practical point of view, let's look at the most common movement in BJJ: shrimping. When do you breathe in and when do you exhale? If you follow my previous example, your inhalation would be at the beginning of the movement when your chest expands. Your exhalation would be at the end, when your body is bent, like a shrimp.

Another good example would be the inverted position. Imagine laying on your back and bringing your fully extended legs over your head and touching the floor behind you. If you tried to breathe in and hold your breath and then bring your legs over your head, you would be unsuccessful. If you have a little space, try it now. Lay on your back and take a deep inhalation. Hold your 'in breath' as you attempt to bring your legs over your head.

You will find it almost physically impossible because your lungs are inflated which prevents the extension of your legs and folding of your torso.

This is important to note because otherwise you could totally be working against yourself in live training.

The first step is to know how to breathe, next we will discuss when to breathe. I always remind my students, "Jiu-Jitsu doesn't happen under water, so there's no need to hold your breath!" This is my lighthearted attempt at reminding them of the importance of controlled, conscious breathing during practice. Holding your breath and catching your breath are both cut from the same cloth.

When you consciously or unconsciously hold your breath, you're disrupting your bodies natural rhythm and balance. Remember, oxygen is the fuel for our brain and muscles. When you deny yourself air it leads to muscle exhaustion and mental fog. Jiu-Jitsu is a full body and mind martial art. It requires that you're physically and mentally available at all times. The act of holding your breath is often a result of stress and fear. It's the mental act of "bracing yourself for impact." As a result your body begins to lock up and become rigid.

The act of 'catching your breath' is often the result of holding onto your air. This sounds almost paradoxical. How can holding your breath cause you to be out of breath? When you stop breathing it causes huge exertions of air being released all at once. This disrupts your internal balance and causes you to inhale and exhale rapidly. As a result, you temporarily lose control of your breathing and create a sense of panic and stress. This is like when you see someone pop up to their feet at the end of a tough round and are bent over breathing erratically. In some cases they will pace around the room searching for more air. They're literally trying to 'catch their breath.' In your own experience how many times have you heard and uttered the phrase? "Hold on, I need to catch my breath!" As if it were outside of you?

The goal with your breathing is to maintain absolute internal control at all times. When your breath gets completely away from you, it will require rest and recovery to get you back in the game. In the ever-changing dynamic game of BJJ conserving your energy allows for clarity of thinking. You cannot expect yourself to solve complex puzzles when you cannot breathe effectively.

It's nearly impossible to solve difficult challenges like BJJ when you're exhausted and stressed out. When you are desperate for oxygen you simply cannot problem solve successfully. Like we discussed in the section on BJJ and breathing, the first step is being conscious of your breath. Simply pay attention to your breathing during matches. When your breathing starts to become erratic, regain control by taking slow, controlled breaths. If your partner is more experienced, listen to their breath and try to match it. If they too are breathing uncontrollably, try to get your breath back and take advantage of the opportunity.

If you reach a point of no return, take slow deep breaths and repeat this mantra: "*If I can breathe, I am alive. If I'm alive, I can think. If I can think, I can problem solve my way out of anything.*" This conscious act not only replenishes your oxygen supply but also refocuses your mind, thus grounding you in the present moment.

This mantra not only serves as a reminder of your resilience but also underscores the interconnectedness of your breath, your consciousness, and your ability to strategize. Remember, your breath is your life force. You cannot exist without out. Harness it, control it, and let it guide you to a conscious, tactical response, no matter how daunting the challenge may seem.

In the same way that you would practice your breathing technique for a grappling match, you can approach your life in a similar fashion. When you feel the pressure and stress of life (which often feels like being stuck in side control) take moments for deep, conscious breathing. It doesn't have to turn into a full-on meditation session either. You can simply take several deep breaths.

Why does this help? When you take deep breaths it activates the parasympathetic nervous system. What is that you ask? Think of it as the "chill out" system for your body. When you're excited or scared another part of your body, the sympathetic nervous system, causes your heart rate to increase and prepares you to react.

The **parasympathetic nervous system** is referred to as "rest and digest." This is where you conserve energy, are calm and attempt to maintain homeostasis (internal balance). Conversely, the sympathetic nervous system is called "fight or flight." Think of it as your "get ready for action", internal "spidey-sense" mechanism. Your heart beats faster, more blood is sent to your muscles and your breathing becomes more rapid.

So how do we control all of this and make sure our body is having the proper reaction to external situations? We have to always go back to our breath, truly our source of life. When we take deep breaths it activates something called the "vagus nerve." (Not like "Vegas" of Los either, but pronounced in the same way) The vagus nerve is like a computer network system that connects the brain to the heart, lungs and stomach. When you take deep breaths your brain sends signals to these parts of your body to be calm and chill.

Think of the **vagus nerve** as a friend who "talks you off the ledge" in moments of stress and anxiety. In the same way that a true friend would put their hand on your shoulder or speak calmly and supportively to you in times of stress, the vagus nerve functions in a similar way. It's like having a homie inside your body that can speak directly to vital parts of your body. These calming signals help you navigate through times of stress and doubt with grace and poise.

- To improve your breathing, you can schedule "breath breaks" throughout your day. Set an alarm in your phone for conscious breathing sessions. These can be every few hours, or whatever works best for your schedule. The purpose of these sessions is to get away from work, family and routine and focus solely on your breath.

- Set a timer for five minutes. Find a quiet space, close your eyes (not while you're driving please) and focus on deep, conscious breathing. Pay attention to the air coming into your body and then leaving. You can simply visualize a particularly comforting environment like a quiet forest or gentle wave. It's important to invite your new, calming "friend" the vagus nerve to the party. Imagine it sending calming signals throughout your body.

This is a simple, yet powerful tool to align your entire being with a state of balance and harmony. It can improve relationships by teaching us how to respond with empathy and understanding. It can help us in work environments by fostering a better sense of creativity and concentration.

The importance of breath control on and off the mats cannot be understated. By tuning into our breath we are connecting to a part of ourselves that is constant and ever-changing. This can foster a feeling that allows us to feel connected to something larger than ourselves. A higher power, the universe, or just perhaps a deeper understanding of our own existence. "The show must go on", but so to must our breath (well until it doesn't any longer). But we'll save that for another day.

Mission:

Stress management in Jiu-Jitsu is not just about handling pressure during rolls but also about integrating relaxation techniques into daily life. Mindfulness, breathing exercises, and cognitive reframing are essential tools.

Include more structured downtime post-training to allow for mental recovery. Incorporate mindfulness exercises at the beginning or end of sessions to cultivate a calmer approach to training and competition.

Daily mindfulness practice post-training. Use visualization techniques to rehearse responses to stressful situations on the mats, reinforcing a calm and strategic mindset.

Understanding Martial Arts Through Physics

Ever wonder how Jiu-Jitsu becomes such a powerful art form that both a wiry teenager and a seasoned adult can excel equally? The answer lies not just in the techniques but in the very physics that govern every move we make on the mats. This chapter delves into the science behind the art, revealing how principles like angular momentum, dynamics, and force distribution are integral to mastering Jiu-Jitsu.

Angular Momentum: The Dance of Dynamics

In Jiu-Jitsu, every sweep, pass, and transition embodies the principle of angular momentum.

Remember the formula $L = m v r$ - where L stands for angular momentum, m is mass, v is velocity, and r is radius.

This isn't just math; it's the secret recipe that lets smaller practitioners manage bigger opponents. It's all about how you position your body (radius), move it (velocity), and apply your weight (mass). By understanding this, you can make physics work for you.

The Play of Stabilizers: Active vs. Inert

Imagine you're in a side control position; your body acts as an active stabilizer, dynamically adjusting to maintain control and apply pressure. Contrast this with inert stabilizers — parts of your body that remain static, providing a base for your dynamic movements. Balancing these stabilizers is crucial for maintaining position and transitioning smoothly without giving up control.

Force Distribution: The Art of Pressure

Ever felt stuck under a well-executed side control? That's force distribution in action. Effective Jiu-Jitsu isn't about applying maximum force everywhere but about distributing it strategically. By varying pressure points and understanding how and where to apply force, you can control and submit opponents more efficiently, using their resistance against them.

Fluid Dynamics: Flow Like Water

BJJ is as much about flow as it is about fight. Fluid dynamics teaches us to streamline movements to conserve energy — think of it as moving through water. The smoother your movements, the less energy you waste, and the harder it is for opponents to predict and counter your actions. It's about creating paths of least resistance, where you move with, not against, the forces at play.

Elemental Jiu-Jitsu: Air, Water, Fire, Earth

Air (Efficient Breath): Breathing isn't just about keeping you going; it's a tactical tool. Controlled breathing keeps you calm and focused, allowing you to perform under pressure.

Water (Flowing Movement): Be adaptable. Change tactics as seamlessly as water changes its course around rocks.

Fire (Explosive Energy): Know when to explode into action. Timing this right can be the difference between a successful sweep and a missed opportunity.

Earth (Grounded in Leverage): Use the ground as your ally. Leverage is foundational in BJJ, grounding your techniques in stability and strength.

Martial vs. Art: The Dual Nature of Jiu-Jitsu

Martial Attributes — Attributes like strength, speed, and flexibility are your physical toolkit. However, they have diminishing returns. Use them wisely to conserve your energy for when it truly counts.

Artistic Attributes — Leverage, timing, and technique form the soul of Jiu-Jitsu. These aren't just about physicality; they involve understanding the deeper mechanics of movement and reaction, the predictive play of human chess.

Applying Physics to Practice

Understanding the physics behind Jiu-Jitsu enhances not just your physical execution but also your conceptual approach. Every drill, every spar, and every roll is an opportunity to apply these principles. Observe, experiment, and adapt. Remember, Jiu-Jitsu is not just an art or a martial practice; it's a science.

Mission:

Embracing the physics of Jiu-Jitsu doesn't mean becoming a physicist but understanding and utilizing these principles can elevate your practice from technique to mastery. As you train, think about the forces at play, the energy you're using, and how you can make each action more efficient and effective. This understanding transforms good practitioners into great ones, who not only move but think with the curves and flows of Jiu-Jitsu.

The Anatomy of Jiu-Jitsu

Arming yourself with anatomical knowledge transforms you from being merely a practitioner to being a master of your own body. In BJJ, every grip, every move, every escape starts and ends with the understanding of the body's mechanics.

Every warrior knows that the greatest victory is the one that allows you to fight another day. In BJJ, injury prevention is paramount. Understanding the anatomy not only enhances performance but also fortifies the body against common injuries.

Proprioception: often described as the body's "sixth sense," refers to the ability to sense the position, location, orientation, and movement of the body and its parts.

- In BJJ, proprioception enables practitioners to understand their body positioning relative to their opponent without needing to look, allowing for more intuitive and effective responses during rolling or competition.

Joint Mechanics: involves the study of how joints move and bear forces, including aspects like leverage and rotational forces.

- Joints are the very levers and fulcrums that dictate the dance of a fight. Take the shoulder: a ball-and-socket joint designed for mobility over stability, allowing for the extensive range of motion necessary for executing armbars or for a simple shrimp escape (hip joint). Contrast this with the hinge-like structure of the elbow or the complex workings of the knee—each joint has its strategic function, and knowing how to engage these can turn your body into a more effective grappling machine.

Muscle Groups Engagement: how different muscle groups function, focusing on their roles in movement and stabilization.

- In Jiu-Jitsu, your muscles are the engine behind the techniques. The quadriceps and hamstrings drive explosive takedowns, while the core muscles—not just your abs, but also your obliques and lower back—stabilize your body through every roll and sweep. Enhanced strength and flexibility in these groups amplify your performance and resilience, turning good grapplers into great ones.

Rickson Gracie once said, *"In the fight, only one person can be comfortable. Your job is to transfer the comfort from your opponent to you."*

Importance of Spinal Alignment and Head Position:

- Proper spinal alignment is crucial in BJJ for maintaining balance, executing movements effectively, and preventing back injuries, particularly in moves that involve twisting and bending.

- The head, heavy and pivotal, when moved correctly, can dictate the balance of both fighters, leveraging the vestibular system, which keeps you upright and oriented. Mastery of the vestibular system's functions aids BJJ athletes in maintaining balance during dynamic movements and in situations where they cannot rely on visual cues, enhancing control in unstable positions.

Mission:

- Understanding joint mechanics helps BJJ practitioners apply techniques more efficiently and safely, maximizing leverage and minimizing risk of injury.

- Knowledge of muscle function helps practitioners optimize the use of strength and endurance, allowing for more effective application of force and resistance during techniques.

- Proper alignment of your spine and head ensures optimal balance and control, which can significantly impact your ability to maintain or escape positions.

- Effective head positioning is essential for protecting the neck during rolls and for influencing the balance and posture of both the practitioner and their opponent.

Warm up properly, respect the limits of your joints, maintain flexibility, and always—always—prioritize technique over brute strength. Proper technique is not just about effectiveness; it's about safety. We don't just train our moves; we train our bodies to be smarter, sharper, and always one step ahead. Now let's roll!

Nagging Injuries

Nobody wants surgeries and other terrible injuries. But sometimes it's those annoying, nagging injuries and can be the most inconvenient. You know, that one finger or toe that drives you crazy. Here we will discuss the most common and disruptive injuries and what you can do about them.

Recognizing the signs of common training injuries can save you from long-term setbacks. Listen to Your Body and go 20% less then you're capable of. Pain is a warning signal. If a movement hurts, stop and assess. Your body communicates its limits and needs—heed its call.

ARITA Method: Dr. Gabe Merkin, the founder of the RICE method, now advocates for the ARITA approach—Active Recovery Is The Answer. Instead of complete rest, engage in gentle, active movements that do not exacerbate the pain. This promotes faster healing and maintains mobility.

Mat burn -

Every new white belt knows this pain. There's nothing worse than a friction burn tearing the skin clear from your foot. The problem isn't the initial trauma, but the constant re-tearing of the epidermis. Every time you train it becomes a problem. If you notice mat burn on your body, clean it and cover it immediately. If you return to training, you will want to cover it with gauze and tape. To get through the first few weeks of mat burn, keep it covered in class. (Ace bandage, gauze, sock, sometimes shoes if allowed) The key is to let it heal and not keep tearing it open.

Sore throat from a misplaced choke -

This is why you tap early and often. Don't wait on collar strangulations. Your partners arm often passes by your trachea which can cause trauma. If you're drilling chokes then ask your partner to keep it chilled out and not to crank anything. This is very common when you practice guillotine chokes. If your throat hurts try using an herbal tea for relief. (Or just be more careful and tap early)

Turf toe -

The name comes from injuries that were sustained from playing American football on artificial turf. This is caused by a hyperextension of the big toe, usually caused by planting it on the floor during BJJ training. I have personally dealt with this on and off for years. I can attest that it is incredibly painful and shouldn't be trifled with. The problem with this injury is that it's very easy to re-injure. If you're prone to turf toe you can try training with wrestling shoes. The key is to let it heal fully. You can also try taping it, but if it's chronic, have it looked at by a a real doctor, not the academy bro's.

Tennis and golfers elbow (tendonitis) -

With tennis elbow, the outside tendons are affected. With golfers elbow, the tendons on the inside of the elbow are affected. This is typically an overuse injury from gripping, twisting and turning your wrist and arm. I have also had challenges with tennis elbow. I found that acupuncture was very effective in treating it. Massage and myofascial release are also purported to be a very effective form of treatment for tendinitis. The "Theraband Flexbar", available on Amazon is also excellent for treatment. The "flexbar" has accompanying exercises that you follow that work very well to alleviate the discomfort and strengthen the area.

Rib injuries -

Never train through rib injuries as they can become serious. Always seek medical advice, especially if you're experiencing pain or discomfort. Rib injuries can be common in BJJ from a partners pressure or twisting your own body. By warming up properly and maintaining a strong core you can prevent rib trauma. If you're coming back from such an injury consider wearing a padded compression shirt or rib protection. Be sure to let your partners know that you're just coming off an injury. This is one of those injuries that you can easily re-injure and further set yourself back.

Chronic finger pain -

If you train in the gi you may experience challenges with finger health. This is especially true if you like to play a lot of spider guard. The hook grip in particular is a nightmare on your finger joints. That's why you often see the top set of knuckles looking the worst on someone who has trained with the gi for years. Try to limit your use of the spider guard position and alternate to using a pistol grip (versus a hook grip). The pistol grip is better on your hands because you can easily release it at anytime.

I also find that lapel chokes are overall better on finger and hand health. (strangles and gripping that utilizes the bottom tail of the gi - versus the top lapels near the neck) With the tail you can release your hand from the choke safely when needed. Sometimes with a collar choke, especially the baseball grips version, your hands and fingers can take a beating. Whereas with the tail you can easily let go of the choke whenever needed. A hand massage can be helpful in releasing any tightness. I also recommend a "Paraffin wax bath" for your hands. Amazon sells a "Therabath, Professional Thermotherapy" Paraffin wax bath. These are recommended by physical therapists for the treatment of arthritis pain.

Cauliflower fingers -

Much like the ear version. This is caused by the build up of fluid in the finger joints that hardens and causes pain and stiffness. Massage and myofascial release can help. What to do? Improve gripping and don't fight holds to the death. Taping fingers can be helpful. Warm-up your hands and fingers before training, and stretch them regularly.

Repetitive joint injuries -

The key word here is "repetitive." If you're taking all of your joint supplements and you're still experiencing problems. It's probably from something that you're doing during training that's causing it. More often than not, it's from too much of one thing over and over. You have to be extra mindful about how you drill joint locks. You can't practice until it hurts. I cringe when I overhear this conversation from two new white belts drilling an arm bar. "Nope… don't feel it, keep going… more pressure. AWW-WW!!!!! Right there that's it!" The constant jarring pressure on your joints is not healthy or sustainable.

You don't need to "feel a move" for every rep that's completed. You can gently drill without killing each other. Also be sure to tap early when drilling joint locks. I tell my own students, "I don't even want to see you tapping during drilling. Just go to the end of the technique and stop. There's no need to traumatize your body over and over during practice, that's not part of the technique."

Even when you're rolling you can play "catch and release." It's a lot like fishing. You catch the submission, but realize it before they tap and keep going. You don't catch the fish, unhook it, stomp on it and throw it back dead. You want that fish to grow even bigger for another day of fishing.

Lower back pain can be utterly frustrating. But if you follow some basic advice it can be prevented. As always be sure to warm up properly. Never roll or train cold. If you're late for class (purple belts) always make time to properly loosen the muscles you will be using. Work on your posture outside of class. Especially if you work at a desk all day. If this is the case, find micro-moments throughout your work day to stand, stretch and move your body. I have found all of the following to work well for lower back pain: foam rolling, acupuncture, massage / myofascial release work, hot epsom salt bath, daily stretching, strengthening your core.

Neck and shoulder pain -

As always a good warm up is ideal. But it's equally important to cool down as well. At the end of an open mat or rolling session, spend 10-15 minutes stretching the shoulder and neck. Door frame stretches are great. Corner stretches also work well - Face the corner of the room (your body pressed against the corner), extend each arm behind you, conforming to the angle of each wall.

The Iron Neck is an incredible piece of equipment to help strengthen and recover the neck, shoulders, spine and back. Using it has personally helped me add strength and recover from old injuries. I give it my highest recommendation. But it's not just about the neck as it strengthens the entire chain: neck, shoulders and down the back.

Knee injuries -

Whenever someone asks me about knee injuries I always reply with, "Are you taking your joint supplements?" I have struggled with knee pain over the course of my martial arts journey. When I consistently take my joint supplements, the pain subsides. When I do not, the pain returns. This is how I know that they work. For joint health I recommend at a minimum what I call "The trifecta" - Krill oil, collagen, and a solid joint supplement.

Krill oil -

Some studies indicate that krill oil can "significantly decrease arthritis symptoms and inflammation." The omega-3 fatty acids found in high concentrations in krill oil can help lubricate joints. Some studies show that they may also slow the progression of osteoarthritis by stopping cartilage from breaking down.

Collagen -

The most abundant protein in your body. It is used to make connective tissue. It's also great for nails, skin, hair and bone health. It can be purchased at any health food store in a powder form.

Joint Supplement -

For a joint supplement to be effective it needs to do the following: reduce inflammation, promote cartilage synthesis (the system for producing more cartilage), and provide the building blocks for connective tissues. Look for these top four ingredients: Glucosamine, Chondroitin, Methylsulfonylmethane (MSM), Omega-3 Fatty Acids. These can often be found in one pill or you can take them separately.

"Loose hips, make better knees!" This is my personal mantra. In spite of the fact that as a teen I was told I would have a lifetime of knee problems.

But here I am after 40 plus years of martial arts and NO KNEE SURGER-IES! I discovered that in my early 40's that if my hips were opened, my knees were no longer compromised. What does it mean to have "opened hips?" This is a term that is often used in yoga and pilates to describe someone who has achieved a high degree of hip flexibility free from pain or discomfort. For me, I can fully stretch my hips without any pain. It's kind of like being able to do "the splits" but with your hips.

When my hips were tight it caused me to load more body weight on my knees. By loosening and opening my hip flexors and hip adductors I reduced the load significantly. I went from not being able to sit in the seiza position (kneeling and sitting with my butt on my heels). Now I can not only sit in this position, but I can lay all the way back with my shoulders on the floor. This is important to note because with open hips, my knees are under less stress and strain.

The hip flexors and hip adductors are important for the movement and stability of our hips. They are involved in a variety of movements, including bending and sitting as well as walking and running. These muscles can influence our general posture, movement mechanics, and even create pain or discomfort when they are tight or unbalanced. In addition to saving your knees, loose hips allow you to physically do more complex movements pain free and with fluidity.

<u>Here are my favorite hip opening stretches:</u>

- Pigeon pose (yoga)

- Frog pose (similar to yoga but with modifications) - Perform two sets. One with your toes turned away, and one with the big toes turned towards each other.

- Happy baby pose (yoga)

- Old school seated butterfly stretch - Sit with your bottoms of your feet together and knees bent to form "butterfly wings." Hold the feet in pace as you slowly lower your head to your toes.

- Lizard pose (yoga)
- Seated forward bend - Sit with your legs extended and straight. Keep your knees flat to the floor and toes pointed upward. Slowly bend forward and reach for your ankles or toes.

I also strongly recommend **walking backwards**. Yes, you read that right, walking backwards. I discovered the wonders of walking in reverse from "The Knees over toes guy", Ben Patrick. He has written a wonderful book called "Knee Ability Zero." In it he outlines several great exercises and stretches for those with "zero knee ability." Walking in reverse, also known as "retro walking" has been practiced by various cultures for centuries. I have been walking backwards for some time now and can attest to the benefits. Because your toes strike the ground first (versus the heel when walking forward) you have less impact on your knee joints. This is vital for people who suffer from knee pain. They often fall into a trap where the muscles surrounding the knees are weak. But they cannot exercise due to the intense pain. Walking backwards will allow you to build muscle, pain free! Walking backwards in a pool is also highly recommended.

Cauliflower ear is caused by blunt trauma to the ear. The name comes from the bumpy appearance left by scarring that looks like a cauliflower. It has been seen in boxing, rugby and wrestling. The condition has been recognized since the ancient Roman and Greek warriors. In modern BJJ circles some people think of it as a battle scar that was earned through combat. Others think that it's ugly. While some even say it's a sign of "poor technique."

I think some ears are just more susceptible than others and it also has to do with how you grapple. If you're a heavy pressure passer you'll probably experience more ear trauma. Whereas a guard player might be more protected. There are however some preventative measures that can be taken if you're concerned about developing cauliflower ear.

Wrestling ear guards can be temporarily used while your ear is healing. Wearing them ongoing can be uncomfortable and annoying to your training partners. They tend to be bulky and make hearing difficult.

Magnets are sometimes used as part of the healing process. After the fluid is drained, two magnets are put on each side of the ear. The magnets apply a steady, gentle pressure to the area, which keeps fluid from building up again and helps the body heal. Bandages or tape can be used to hold the magnets in place.

Most cauliflower ear heals up without much scarring. But if your ear is extremely swollen it's worth having it looked at by a medical professional. Always stay away from fellow students offering to drain your ear with a syringe. It's probably not the safest and most sterile way of doing it. Don't let it go untreated if it's extremely swollen. The ear can permanently close and make hearing difficult. Here's my cautionary tale: I once knew a guy who had terrible, untreated cauliflower ear. It got so bad that his ear closed up entirely. He would take drinking straws and cut them real small and smoosh it in his ear to help his hearing. Don't become that guy.

Mission:

Seek new solutions to old problems.

Do your own research. Set time aside to specifically focus what you can do when pain strikes.

Learn about supplements and how they can help you.

Do less than you're capable of, staying in the game is what is the most important. Don't let speed, strength, or being over stretched slow you down.

Keith Owen Tribute

Professor Keith Owen was a 4th Degree Black Belt under the world renowned Master Pedro Sauer. He dedicated his life to continuing the legacy of his teachers Jiu-Jitsu and founded the Team Rhino Association based out of Boise, ID.

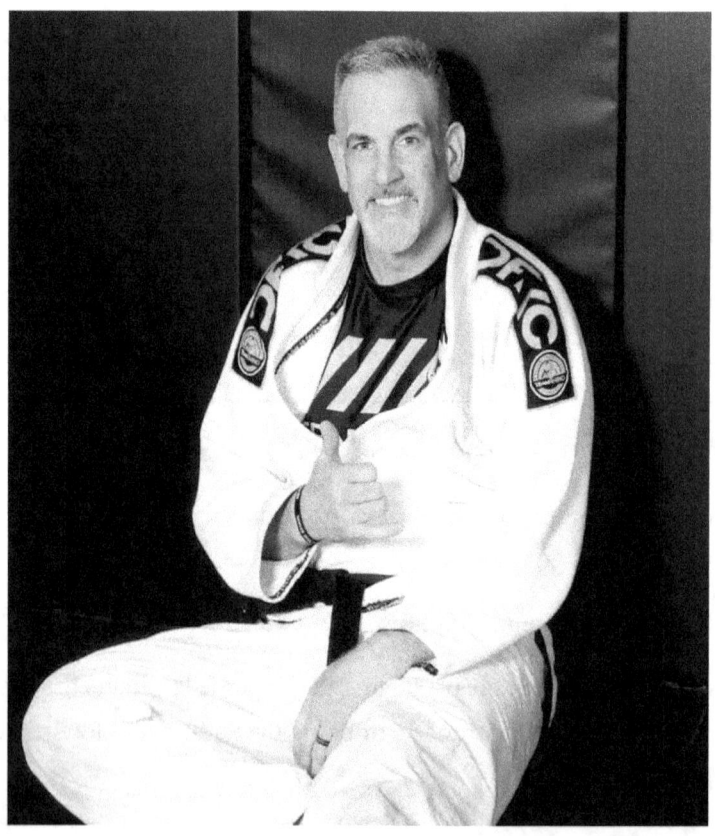

Intel:

Nowadays we are inundated with BJJ techniques online. Sometimes I even need to tell my YouTube algorithm to calm down! Even I need a break from BJJ from time to time. In the early days there was little to no content. But my favorite resource back then was always "Submission-101" with Keith Owen.

Here was this larger than life BJJ teacher who was also the same age as me and shared that same old school vibe. His teachings resonated with me and has impacted my BJJ to this day.

I have never physically met Keith in person but we were friends online. He would always pop onto a BJJ After 40 post and drop a knowledge bomb and blow everyone away... *then disappear like a true ninja.*

I always felt Keith's support both in front of and behind the BJJ scene. He would send me a random kind message every so often and make my week. Like on New Year's Eve when he sent me this amazing message that I saved:

"Happy New Year Mike and I appreciate your contribution to Jiu-Jitsu. You are making it better. 😊 #justsayin"

This was my last interaction with him and just a few months before he unexpectedly passed away.

When I heard of Keith's passing it stung deeply. He was an inspiration to me and so many others.

We were the same age and now that a few years have passed I feel even more compelled than ever to leave Jiu-Jitsu as Keith would have liked it.... *Better.*

-Mike Bidwell

Preventing Injuries During Training

If you're just getting started in BJJ and haven't worked out in years, you may want to consider training 2-3 class days per week. When we first begin our BJJ journey there's a lot of excitement and we may want to train every day. Unfortunately its just not realistic. It's okay to start one way, and finish in another way. It may be two days per week for now, but you can gradually increase as your body adapts to the intensity of BJJ. Ultimately, find a rhythm that works for you.

One of my hard and fast rules is to ALWAYS warm up properly. If you're a purple belt this may be a tough one for you. As the lore goes, "blue belts quit" and "purple belts skip warm ups!" Don't do either.

Warm ups: Try to always be on time for class to not miss the warm ups. I believe they are crucial for an over 40 student. As you age, your body needs more adjustment time. You can't just jump from a twenty minute car ride to having your legs thrown over your head! Your body (and mind) may need a second to adjust to the new environment and conditions. That's the purpose of a warm-up, to gradually increase blood flow and prepare your body for BJJ practice.

A good warm up should combine the following:

- Light cardio - jogging or walking backwards (awesome for those with knee stability issues).

- Mobility movements - Move the way you will move for BJJ practice. I like exercises that put you close to the ground and you can use it for leverage in your movements. Example: Moving like an animal (gorilla walks, alligator crawls, snake movement, rolls - forward / backwards, shrimping, break falls, technical stand up, etc.)

- Solo drills - Moving on the mats and simulating the mechanics of a submission, sweep or reversal. If you like triangles like me, then move your hips and legs for your favorite submissions.

- Body weight exercises - Functional movements are the key. Examples: Push ups, pull ups, air squats, lunges, planks, back bridge.

- Stability ball - You know that big inflatable ball that sits in the corner of most academies? Well it's perfect for getting loose and prepared for training. You can use it to stretch your spine and core muscles. It can also be used to replicate a real partner for guard passing, positional control, back takes, etc.

- Partner drills - The key here is to set perimeters so you can keep yourselves in check. DON'T ever roll cold. You also don't want partner drills to escalate into live rolling. Perimeters - Catch and release (never tap your partner when you move, but go for submissions with a catch it and let it go mentality) You can both agree to move at 20 - 30% speed and try to hit every main position (guard, side, mount, back). Eyes closed is another option to slow the game down and focus on technique. Agree that both partners will close their eyes during the roll. Be mindful of walls and coffee tables! (In other words, don't try this at home, at least not near any valuables)

- Grappling dummy - For the first time ever, grappling dummies are affordable. Of course they can never replace a real human partner, but they can be a good training tool. (And someone to converse with, when the mood strikes) You can drill most techniques with some degree of success. They're also excellent to throw a gi on and collar choke. (Plus no whining that "You're squeezing my jaw!" If you have one at home you can always drill to a light sweat before you leave for class. Having a head start on warm ups can be helpful.

Now that you're properly warmed up and ready to roll, it's vital that you prioritize building good technique and Jiu-Jitsu comprehension. One of the most common ways to get injured is through poor technique. When your mechanics are wrong, you put yourself and your partners at risk for injury. Good technique is your responsibility. The scuba diver doesn't trounce on the coral reef and destroy it for the next diver. Leave yourself and your partner better than you found them.

Be sure to know your audience. You're about to roll with someone you don't know. How can you determine what skill level they're at? In gi training their belt color should give you your first clue. Next look at their size and approximate age. As a 40 plus roller it's perfectly acceptable to set a few guidelines before the roll. You just have to make sure you respect and honor the rules you've set.

You can't say, "Hey let's roll light, then go full ADCC on someone" I like to build the rhythm of the match as it progresses. I always remind my partners, "Let's start light and build on it." That allows you both to adjust to the intensity as it happens. Versus being thrown in and you both are fighting for survival. Remember a good BJJ technique is built from leverage, timing and technique - Not Strength alone.

Leverage is how we use "strength" when we have no power. It's a mechanical process, which is why it's so powerful. It doesn't require toughness or grit, it's a technology. Just like your phone doesn't care if you make a weird face to unlock it. The technology of BJJ is absent of your emotional state. You don't need to add any "UMPH" - the technique when done correctly, stands alone. Like the aforementioned phone, the technology also will not work when done incorrectly no matter how mad or frustrated you get. If you try to unlock your phone with the wrong code, it won't work. It reacts to a set of predetermined commands. You can get as mad as you want. If you keep putting in the wrong number it won't unlock. In fact, eventually it will lock you out! The point is that you need to understand how to properly utilize the technology of Jiu-Jitsu as it relates to your body and your partners. Getting mad, upset, frustrated, amped up, psyched up or psyched out, etc. won't help your cause. If anything, they will dramatically slow your progress.

When you begin to develop good technique you rely less on strength, speed and athleticism. Yes, they will support the technique. But they aren't the technique alone. Think of it this way. If this were a dinner, the technique is the main course. Whereas strength, speed and athleticism are the seasoning. You don't dump on the seasonings. You add just enough to make it palatable and maybe a little tastier. You don't drown in flavor. Remember, strength and speed have a diminishing return. The more you use them, the less you'll have available. Every time you use strength or speed there's an immediate recovery period.

Go ahead and do push-ups until you're tired. After sometime you'll reach failure and need to recover in order to do more. Otherwise you risk injury. Focus on good form and reserve your strength and speed for when you really need it!

Mission:

Stress management in Jiu-Jitsu is not just about handling pressure during rolls but also about integrating relaxation techniques into daily life. Mindfulness, breathing exercises, and cognitive reframing are essential tools.

Include more structured downtime post-training to allow for mental recovery. Incorporate mindfulness exercises at the beginning or end of sessions to cultivate a calmer approach to training and competition. Daily mindfulness practice post-training. Use visualization techniques to rehearse responses to stressful situations on the mats, reinforcing a calm and strategic mindset.

The Team: Having fun with "The BJJ Cast of Characters"

Like any hobby or endeavor, BJJ is filled with a wild cast of characters. In this section we laced a little humor into the conversation. But some version of all of these personalities and stereo types exits within the world of grappling. You will definitely be able to spot a few, hopefully it's not you. In this section I used the word "guy" to describe these characters, but these certainly can apply to anyone.

"Stinky guy" - You know the guy who smells like bad onions? You cringe when he says, "hey let's roll!" It's okay to nicely tell him that his hygiene needs an upgrade. But you have to handle it in a kind manner. Instead of saying, "You have terrible B.O." Say something like, "It might be time to retire that gi." (Or spats, rash guard, etc.) "I noticed your gi smells a little funky." You can share with them the section in this book on stripping down your gi. Remember foul smells are indicative of the presence of bacteria and micro-organisms. If you're uncomfortable saying something, talk to your professor about the situation.

"No rash guard under the gi guy" - Sometimes this too can be 'stinky guys' problem. The old school way was to wear just a gi top, bottoms and belt with no rash guard under the kimono. Very similar to the practice of Judo. Some BJJ associations even have practitioners only wear white gi's with no rash guard underneath (except for females of course).

There's a memorable scene from the movie "Along Came Polly" when the main character Reuben Feffer (played by Ben Stiller) plays a pick up game of basketball with his friend Sandy Lyle (Philip Seymour Hoffman - R.I.P.), and a group of other guys. Sandy who is out of shape and sweating profusely, rubs his bare sweating chest against Feffer's face. The cringe-worthy scene is shown up close and in slow motion to emphasize this stomach churning moment. This is exactly how it feels inside 'no rash guard under the gi guys' guard.

"Too much taped finger guy" - This guys hands look like he's one of the wounded coming off a civil war era battlefield. Every finger, knuckle and joint is covered in tape. He may even have very specific brands, colors and taping styles he uses. By the end of an open roll, you'll likely find his tape remnants strewn about the mats.

"Never stops sweating guy" - This dude sweats like a firehose. If he's self-aware he will have a towel. Unfortunately that minimal piece of cloth is usually too small for the job. It's like bringing a dish towel to a tropical rain storm. I know because I too am a "sweater." I always have a second gi top on hand, and always shower before I leave the dojo.

"Spats only guy" - He shows up to no-gi in almost no clothing. He generally wears just a set of spats (compression pants) and a rash guard. (No shorts over the spats) This is generally okay if he's not "never stops sweating guy" too (which is often the case). Rolling with him can feel like you're trying to grab a wet, slimy fish.

"Never washes their belt, or gi guy" *see stinky guy - First off, there's no excuse to not wash your gi after training. Like I stated before I sweat profusely when I train. I couldn't imagine trying to put that wet mess of a gi back on again the next day! Always wash your gi right after training. Avoid letting the sweat dry into the gi. I always recommend washing your belt regularly. Don't worry you won't wash away the knowledge. Remember, your belt is like any other part of your gi and isn't immune to bacteria.

"Aways injured guy" - He comes to class every day but can't understand why he's always hurt? When you roll with him and ask, "How are you doing" You'll get a page long list of injuries. He might start the match by saying, "Watch out for my shoulder it's a little tweaked, also my backs been tight and my neck is jacked, but other than that I should be good!" You're left thinking, what am I left to grapple with, your big toe?

"Talks too much during rolling guy (aka the commentator)" - The reason people talk during rolling can be a sign of nervousness or insecurity. This is especially true of novices. I always remind my own students that at some point you need to 'outgrow' this habit. If they persist and it gets annoying, politely ask if you can both roll silently.

"Tells you, How to submit them as you submit them guy" - If you train long enough you'll definitely have this experience. You're rolling hard, you make the transition into a submission, you elevate your hips for the inevitable tap and…. You hear your partners voice underneath you say, "Good job, now elevate your hips!" They are suddenly coaching you through the rest of the move you got on them while they were previously resisting?! This one can be particularly annoying. The best blunt response is, "You should be more concerned about the tap and not coaching me!" The not-so blunt response could be, "I've got the rest of it, thanks!" The reality is that they're having this response out of their own insecurity and embarrassment. At some point they need to evolve past this if they want to truly be successful at BJJ.

"Asks to go light, but always goes hard guy" - You get ready to start a match and your partner makes the verbal gesture, "Let's go light!" (Famous last words by the way) The second your fists bump, he jumps on you like a hungry hyena. Always be leery of this guy as you might get caught with the occasional elbow and knee too.

"Let's just flow guy" - This can be another variation of the tactics used by, "Asks to go light, but always goes hard guy." Don't fall for his trickery. If you know he goes hard, then always be prepared for it. If you don't know someone, always expect they'll be a little crazy. Even if they say, "let's just flow", or "lets go light."

"The move collector guy" - This dude has every instructional video ever made and can also be referred to as "YouTube guy" too. (Most often they are at blue belt level) The move collector guy thinks he can teach every move as if he was the person on the video initially instructing it. He may even have memorized the verbiage and script from the videos too. The challenge with this fella is that he can demonstrate the move, but can rarely if ever, do it during 'live' rolling. *Warning* he can transform into "Tells you how to submit them after you submit them guy" when you're grappling with him.

"I only have one gi guy" (*see stinky guy) - One gi simply is not enough for anyone training in BJJ. It also leaves the temptation to not wash it between training, which is never a good idea. Invest in a second or third gi, even if it's a cheaper one.

"Drives to and from class in his gi and belt guy" - I understand the need to show up on time with all your gear in tow. But you're not five years old either, you don't need to wear your jammies to the movie theater in case you fall asleep. Maybe just wear the gi pants and rash guard and carry the gi jacket with the belt tied around it. (A much better look) Plus were you planning on driving home in a wet gi?

"Underhanded compliment guy" - Have you ever tapped someone and they say afterwards, "What do you weigh? You're really strong!" Or for smaller players, "Wow you are really squirmy!" Those are not real compliments. They're generally excuses for them not doing well. They think they're saying something "nice." But really it's an excuses disguised an underhanded compliment. But you could technically take it as a compliment because you're tapping them, which says everything about your game. At the end of the day, don't take it too personal.

You will come across all kinds of different people and personalities through the practice of BJJ. As much as we poked fun here, it's truly what makes Jiu-Jitsu so special. The vast array of people from all different backgrounds. The diversity that is present in BJJ is rarely seen in other pursuits. This is a testament to the universal appeal of the gentle art. Each individual school represents a tribe that is part of a bigger collection of practitioners. The sense of community coupled with the opportunity for personal growth is what attracts so many to BJJ.

Mission:

Understand and respect the traditional practices of different BJJ associations, but also advocate for modern hygiene standards.

Partake in cultivating a supportive, inclusive, and enjoyable training environment by recognizing, understanding, and positively engaging with the diverse personalities that populate the BJJ community..

Debriefing Assessment:

Training in BJJ demands discipline not just in practice but in maintaining hygiene, which is crucial for a healthy training environment. Assess your daily training routines and hygiene practices. How diligently do you follow protocols like washing your gi after each session, and maintaining personal cleanliness to prevent infections?

Injuries are inevitable in any physical sport, and how we deal with them can significantly impact our training continuity and effectiveness. Reflect on your approach to handling injuries—do you rest adequately, seek appropriate medical advice, and adhere to recovery protocols? Additionally, evaluate the preventive measures you incorporate into your training to minimize injury risks.

The social environment within a BJJ gym plays a crucial role in a practitioner's development. Consider how the dynamics within your gym affect your learning and training. Are there supportive relationships, healthy competition, and a nurturing atmosphere that promotes growth?

Understanding the journey of belts and stripes in BJJ is fundamental to gauging your progress. Reflect on your own progression—how do you perceive your advancement, and what goals do you set for each stage of your journey?

Jiu-Jitsu can be as mentally challenging as it is physically. Assess how you manage stress both on and off the mats. How does the stress of learning new techniques or preparing for competitions affect you, and what strategies do you use to manage it?

Dive into the technical aspects of your training. How well do you understand and apply principles like angular momentum and L.T.T. (Leverage, timing and Technique)? How do these principles reflect in your sparring sessions and technical drills?

Every BJJ gym has a variety of personalities that enrich the training experience. Reflect on the roles you and your fellow gym members play. How do these interactions contribute to a vibrant and dynamic learning environment?

Lastly, it's essential to remember that BJJ is not just about competition and growth but also about enjoyment and community. Evaluate how you balance the rigorous demands of training with having fun and building camaraderie with your peers.

Survival Expert: ARI KNAZAN

2nd degree Black Belt in BJJ
under Keith Owen (deceased)
5th Degree Black Belt in Japanese Jiu-Jitsu (Goshin)
under Soke Steve Hiscoe, Co-Founder of the INVICTUS
Jiu-Jitsu Collective, Founder of "Submissions 101,"
Career Law Enforcement officer

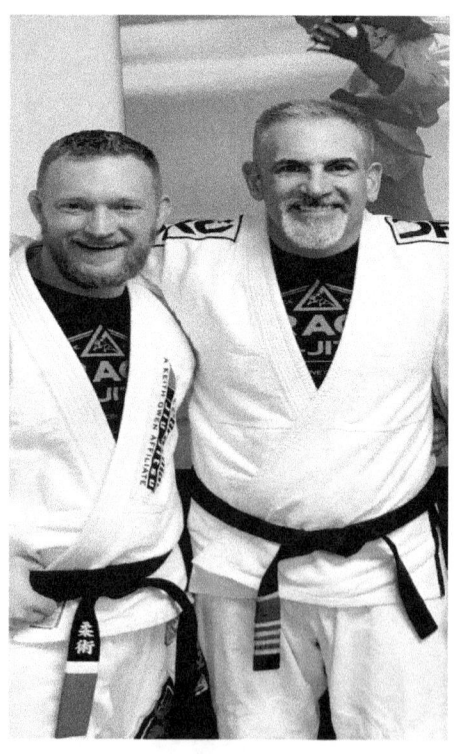

Intel:

I met Ari after the tragic passing of Keith Owen. In every memorial post I read one name came up over and over again... Ari "Kay" Knazan. I quickly learned he was one of Keith's first black belts and of the founders of the iconic "Submissions-101" YouTube channel. He is also a lifelong martial artist and law enforcement officer and trainer and fellow over 40 athlete! He holds a unique perspective for a "real-world" Jiu-Jitsu practice that we can all learn from.

From the Source:

Jiu-Jitsu allows for a scalable use of force option in addition to your tool belt.

If all you know is how to hammer someone in the face, every problem you see becomes a nail. While not every situation requires Jiu-Jitsu, not every situation requires a taser, OC spray or a baton. Jiu-Jitsu won't jam, fail to deploy or misfire.

Police officers need this skill set.

In fact, use of force injuries decrease when you know HOW to control someone.

My driving force has always been a deep desire to learn as much as I can and take that knowledge to teach others. My inspiration comes when I see students have the "ah ha" moments on (and off) the mats. That is my pay off.

I am also deeply connected to my Jiu-Jitsu community and continue to make many new friends. With age (and hopefully maturity), my BJJ journey has changed much since turning 40. After twenty-plus years on the mats in BJJ, the details and possibilities on what this art has to offer have been revealed to me. I'm motivated to understand the little details, the invisible Jiu-Jitsu if you will, that make this art so wonderful.

The most unexpected benefit of practicing BJJ over 40 was the realization of "1% effort." My instructor Keith Owen, used to say "I want to get my output to 1%. I want to fully understand and have all my limbs and body in the perfect place while grappling." Since my body has changed (due to age and injury), I've needed to change how I tackle rolling and moving on the mats. As such, it has moved me down a path where my learning and understanding anatomy and body mechanics has improved. I'm also able to see the limitations.

Listen to those who came before you.

By listening to those who are older and more experienced, it will allow one to circumvent potentially injurious or disastrous consequences on the mats. There is much value to listening to "mat wisdom" as it allows you ways to short cut "dead ends" or "dangerous avenues" during your journey. Seek genuine mentorship from good people. This will pay off tremendously as you make your way through the ranks.

One does not seek legacy. Legacy is what is left after you are gone from this world. I am not looking for accolades and legacy status. I am simply trying to pass on my experience and honor my instructors while doing it. The three "main" people who have influence my martial art career are my Japanese Jiu-Jitsu instructor Steve Hiscoe and my BJJ professor Keith Owen, who passed away in February 2022 and Master Pedro Sauer.

Operations:
Competition

Comprehensive guidance on preparing for and participating in competitions, with personal stories and expert advice on navigating the challenges and maximizing performance.

Scan the QR code for tactics, preparation tips, and psychological strategies for BJJ competitions.

https://www.youtube.com/playlist?list=PLwb5iQup993-uqsRtGhuABEQxIhivMDFu

All the Ins and Outs of Competing

Some schools tend to lean heavily on the competition side and you may feel the pressure to compete. Whether you decide to or not, it should ultimately be up to you. But it's important to seek the guidance of your professor, coaches and training partners. They can provide important feedback that can aid you in your decision. I have personally appreciated the lessons I learned from my time competing in grappling tournaments.

My personal competition experience officially began in 1996 at the very beginning my BJJ journey. Back in the early days there weren't a significant amount of events to participate in. But you could definitely find tournaments if you were willing to travel. It was rare to find one in your city, but the grass roots efforts to grow the sport were taking hold.

Myself and my teammates competed in the very first few N.A.G.A.'s (North American Grappling Association) tournaments held in New England. In fact back then it was still called N.E.G.A. (New England Grapplers Association). We also participated in many of the early "Grappler's Quest" events, along with many others. I wasn't the best competitor back in those days. I wasn't horrible, but I wasn't great either. I almost always finished in 3rd or 4th place, with an occasional runner-up to first place. I had practiced and competed in other martial arts and had done reasonably well in tournaments. However I would often freeze up under the pressure of competing in grappling. It became very mentally challenging for me.

I competed in grappling tournaments sporadically though the mid 90's into the early 2000's with so-so results before stopping altogether. I continued to train in BJJ, but I didn't pursue tournaments again until 2011.

My daughter started training in BJJ when she was three years old. I always told her that if she decided she wanted to compete that I would do it with her. When she turned five years old, she asked me If she could compete, and would I do it with her like I had promised. I agreed but set a goal to lose twenty five pounds to make weight. At the time I was slightly overweight and this would be the perfect impetus to get me on a goal to better health. Plus at this time I had been a brown belt since 2001 and needed to shake up my training if I was ever to receive my black belt.

We both competed and shared first place victories. This was my first time winning first place in a BJJ tournament. Even though this was just a regional event, to me it felt like the world championships. For a guy who never seemed to get past second place it was a more of a mental victory than physical accomplishment. This motivated me to continue competing regularly for the next three years. Competing again created the momentum which put me on a path to better health, the creation of the "BJJ After 40" global community and eventually my black belt promotion in 2014.

I feel like I was a better competitor at 42 than I was at 32 or even 22. With age comes experience and wisdom. As an "older" competitor I was able to stay mentally grounded and not waste crucial energy. Being able to control my emotions and manage my energy was something my younger self couldn't do effectively. With a perspective gained from decades of life behind me I wasn't prone to the nervousness and adrenaline rushes that plagued my earlier performances.

This is the true value of being a 40-plus practitioner, the wisdom from life experiences that can be applied to the present moment. This will allow you to successfully decide whether or not tournaments are for you. I personally gained a ton of directly translatable life experience from my time competing. I gained a deeper sense of trust in myself and my intuition, especially when under stressful conditions. I also made great friendships that I continue to share still today.

The downside is that my body went through physical hell. It wasn't so much the day competing as it was the time leading up to the tournament. I also came from an era where we over-trained and under-prepared.

Yes, I said the correctly. In the early days (pre-2000's) we would literally kill ourselves every day training. This often meant starting every match in an open mat from your feet. We trained full on leg locks, foot locks, neck cranks and just about anything that worked.

We under-prepared by not really preparing at all for said tournament. Nowadays students prep for months or have "training camps" for tournaments. In the "old days" you would hear about a tournament on Thursday and drive five hours on Saturday to compete. There was no real preparation other than going to class.

Through those old experiences I have learned many valuable lessons that, 'I wish I had known then.' Modern BJJ tournaments are very different than the old days. You will often know ahead of time how many people are in your division, who you're competing against and what time your match is scheduled.

If you are considering competing in your first BJJ tournament here's what to expect. The best advice is to go and watch a tournament before competing in one. This gives you the chance to see and experience what competing is like without the risk of getting hurt. I think it's okay to scope it out first and get a feel for what you would be facing. If you go to observe a tournament be sure to watch the master's divisions. It would also be wise to observe competitors of your skill and weight too.

Think of it like a ninja recon mission! Your objective is to observe and gather intel. Pay close attention to the overall flow of the tournament.

How do the brackets progress, how much time is allotted between matches, how are competitors warming up, how do they interact with their coaches, how do they handle wins and losses, and what does the overall energy feel and look like?

Also pay attention to: what types of snacks do competitors consume, how do the rules work, how are points awarded, what kind of gear do competitors wear and bring with them, etc.

When you observe matches look for the following:

- How are points awarded and what do the score cards look like. Is there a digital scoreboard? Is is done manually, etc. Begin to understand and memorize the scoring of techniques.

- What moves are allowed at your skill level and are you familiar with these techniques. If for example you've never done foot locks and they're allowed, this could be put you at a serious risk for an injury.

- How long are matches and how do competitors conserve energy? Do they look tired after matches? Are they breathing heavy and what do the pace of the matches look like? Ask yourself, could you handle rolling at this pace?

- How many competitors are in your division? How many potential matches does it require for you to get first place?

- Are there competitors at your age and weight or would you have to compete in the adult division (under 40) in lieu of masters? If this is the case, do you feel comfortable and safe in those divisions? If you had to enter the adult division, will there also be others your weight as well?

Additional Recon: Use your phone to video as much of the matches and tournament as you can. You can look at previous tournaments in that same circuit and see who won each division. Depending on the belt level, you may even be able to find their matches on YouTube.

Once you decide to compete, what are your next steps?

Stage I: Finding the right tournament and getting signed up

Stage II: Tournament training and preparation

Stage III: Competition day

Stage IV: Afterwards, recovery and reflection

Mission:

Competing is a multifaceted experience that requires mental, physical, and strategic preparation. Tailoring the competition approach to individual strengths and weaknesses is essential.

Enhance strategy training sessions to include more scenario-based drills that mimic competition settings.

Try monthly in-house competitions to simulate the competitive environment. Review and adjust competition strategies based on each event's outcomes.

Stage I : Preparing for Battle

What is the "right" tournament to compete in? There are different tournament circuits you can participate in. Depending on the area where you live and how far you're willing to travel may affect your decision. I would recommend trying to find an event in your immediate area. If you do have to travel, you'll want to plan and budget for a hotel, travel expenses, meals, etc.

If the tournament is five or six hours away, don't be tempted to save money and drive. You'll pay for it by sitting in a cramped up car before you have to compete. If you do decide to drive, take an extra day for traveling so you can recover before the event.

Let's compare bigger national tournaments versus regional events. Both offer advantages and disadvantages for participants. If you compete in an I.B.J.J.F. event you'll have to pre-register before the tournament date. The plus side is you'll know ahead of time exactly how many competitors you'll potentially face and what time you're competing. The downside is the rules are very strict for everything, including the gi and gear you wear. If you don't have any competitors or they don't show up, you still get a medal. This is referred to "winning by default." I.B.J.J.F. tournaments are also more costly as well.

In regional tournaments you can register the day of the event. If you don't have competitors your age they'll often move things around to find someone to compete against you (no winning by default), or offer to let you compete in the "adult" division. (Under 40 division) The downside is that you'll often sit around for sometime waiting for your match to begin. If you move to the adult division, it doesn't come without some risks. *You'll be facing younger, faster opponents in the adult division and this should be taken into consideration. Once you know which event you'll be competing in, you'll want to pick your division. They're broken down by experience (belt level), weight and age. With regional tournaments you generally get to weigh-in the day before, whereas with the I.B.J.J.F. you step on the scale and go right to your match.

If you're close to making your weight it might be advantageous to find an event where you weigh-in the day before. You don't want to starve your-self to make weight and then have to compete without recovering the lost weight back. If you weigh-in early, you'll have plenty of time for the proper recovery of fluids. As a 40-plus competitor it doesn't make sense to do moderate to significant weight-cuts. It's not safe and you'll probably just deplete your energy and not perform well. I've even had experiences where I cut weight and then got to the tournament and they didn't have anyone my weight to compete against. I was now exhausted from losing weight and the only guy they could find was someone a weight class higher than me. I ended up doubly screwing myself!

You're not competing to be the next ADCC World Champion so don't put your body or yourself in these unnecessary and potentially dangerous situations. Remember, your primary goal is to enjoy the sport and grow as a person, not put your health at risk for the sake of a medal. You want to compete fully hydrated and at your natural, healthy weight, with optimal energy levels. The dangers of weight cutting can consist of: dehydration, low energy levels, slower recovery and increased risk of injury. It's best to get yourself to a healthy weight and start from there.

Gi versus No-Gi. Should you compete in one or both, or does it matter?

Some tournaments are gi and some are no-gi, while others offer both. The opportunity to complete in both can be an invaluable experience. But keep in mind that often times the rules can be different for each, so research them before deciding. Look over the list of techniques that are allowed and make sure you're familiar with them. Also be okay with just doing one of the two divisions if you get there and don't have the energy levels to participate in both. You don't want to learn what a bicep slicer is by tapping to it, so always familiarize yourself with all the allotted techniques.

Mission:

Choosing the right tournament involves understanding the competitive landscape and aligning it with personal goals and readiness.

Instructors can develop a clearer guideline for students to assess when they are competition-ready and which tournaments are best suited for their skill levels.

Create a decision matrix for choosing tournaments based on individual goals, current skill level, and logistical considerations.

Stage II: The Heat of Competition

Stay consistent with your training. Try not to miss any classes and give yourself sixty days to prepare for the event. Anything longer and you'll peak out too soon. If the timetable is shorter you might feel mentally and physically underprepared.

Adding weight training and conditioning to your routine can help you build your strength and confidence. But don't over complicate things, keep it simple. You can add two days of weight training with two additional days of conditioning.

Interval training, also know as "**H.I.I.T.**", or **High Intensity Interval Training** is excellent for BJJ athletes. The idea behind this type of workout is to perform high intensity anaerobic exercises followed by short recovery periods. This type of interval training has been around for a very long time, gaining popularity at various times. I love it for BJJ because it mimics the intense bursts of energy and brief moments of recovery that are characteristic of grappling matches. I also like that this type of workout can be done fairly quickly and requires no real equipment.

Here's some examples of interval training sessions modified for BJJ. With this type of workout always push yourself with each exercise, but while listening closely to your body. Be sure to spend 5-10 minutes properly warming up your body. Finish your session with a 5-10 minute cool down stretch. Always keep yourself properly hydrated during and after your training.

*Be smart and listen to your body as you're in charge!

Beginners - Intermediate

Workout #1 Full body:

Air squats - 20 seconds, rest 10 seconds

Push ups - 20 seconds (modify where you need to), rest 10 seconds

Mountain climbers - 20 seconds, rest 10 seconds

Jumping Jacks - 20 seconds, rest 10 seconds

Planks - 20 seconds, rest 10 seconds

Repeat for a cycle of 4-5 rounds followed by a cool down stretch.

Workout #2 Full body:

Kettlebell swing - 20 seconds, rest 10 seconds (if you don't have a kettlebell modify with burpees)

Jump rope - 20 seconds, rest 10 seconds (If you don't have space or can't jump rope, then do "air jump ropes" - simulate the mechanics of jumping rope)

Push ups - 20 seconds, rest 10 seconds

Mountain climbers - 20 seconds, rest 10 seconds

Alternating lunges - 20 seconds, rest 10 seconds

Repeat for a cycle of 4-5 rounds followed by a cool down stretch.

Intermediate - Advanced

Workout #1 Upper body and core:

Push ups - 30 seconds, rest for 10-20 seconds

Mountain climbers - 30 seconds, rest for 10-20 seconds

Tricep dips (use a chair, bench or stability ball) - 30 seconds, rest for 10-20 seconds

Alternating shoulder taps from plank - 30 seconds, rest for 10-20 seconds

Alternate leg air triangle chokes (on your back simulating guard) - 30 seconds, rest for 10-20 seconds

Repeat for a cycle of 4-5 rounds followed by a cool down stretch.

Workout #2 Lower body and core:

Squat jumps - 30-40 seconds, rest for 10-20 seconds

Side planks - 30-40 seconds, rest for 10-20 seconds

Wall sits - 30-40 seconds, rest for 10-20 seconds

Alternate shrimping - 30-40 seconds, rest for 10-20 seconds

Alternate leg air triangle chokes - 30-40 seconds, rest for 10-20 seconds

Repeat for a cycle of 4-5 rounds followed by a cool down stretch.

You can create variables by shortening the rest periods to make it more challenging. You can also interchange the exercises between each workout based on your needs or to just mix it up. As always, consult with your physician before starting a new exercise program.

Functional exercises and drills:

The most important goal through your tournament preparation is to stay 100% injury-free. If you can prepare yourself properly and then enter the event feeling great and in peak condition, you will be a lot further ahead of many other competitors. This is more of a significant achievement than one might think. To be able to compete at your optimal best, pain free, with little to no limitations on performance is the ultimate objective.

Remember, the main adversary will not be on the day of the tournament but everything leading up to it. An effective training camp is one that gets you to the tournament in the best shape possible, mentally, physically, and technically, without any nagging injuries. This requires a mindful approach that balances tough training while respecting your bodies limits.

The best tournament advice I ever received was this, "Save something for the day of the event!" In other words, don't push yourself so hard that you literally have nothing left to compete with. It's tempting to want to propel yourself over the edge while preparing. However, it's better to take yourself to the edge and save the rest for the day of the event.

Another vital part of your preparation will be practicing drills and scenarios that will build your confidence, intuition and reactivity, essentially preparing you for any situation that might arise during the tournament. If you have dealt with it in training, it doesn't become foreign and stressful during competition. Using different prep drills will strengthen your intuition, allowing you to "feel" and anticipate what your partner is going to do, instead of consciously trying to make vital decisions in the heat of combat.

In this section we will expand on the tournament prep by sharing different drills you can use in training to help you prepare for your tournament experience. With drilling the goal is to NOT win the drill, but to improve your game. Always make it a collaborative experience with whatever perimeters you both deem necessary.

Positional drills - maintaining offensive control:

Guard -

Have your partner start in your guard and they have to aggressively try to pass while you defend your position. This is similar to the "traditional pass, sweep or submission" where they try to pass and you try to sweep or submit them. In this case they should try to pass in both familiar and unfamiliar ways but with an aggressive intent. You want the drill to make you start to feel more comfortable in uncomfortable situations. Your goal is to maintain positional control or to sweep them, but not to submit them.

Top side control -

You start from the top and choose a side control position (100-kilos, kesa gatame, reverse kesa, etc.). The mission is to maintain top control, while traversing through various side control positions. Your ultimate goal is to get to knee on belly, north south, the far side of the body, etc. Do not advance to mount, stay along the perimeter of their body.

Try to get through -

100-kilos, kesa gatame, reverse kesa, twister side control, north south, knee on the belly. You can attempt to hit all of these or whatever fits into your style or strategy. Your partners job is to aggressively defend from the bottom position. Have them defend in ways that are both familiar and unfamiliar. A little chaos is invited (just don't kill each other). The rhythm of a competition match is very different than rolling with your buddies in class.

*Version #2 - You can have your partner try to recover guard while you're in side control. But with this version if they recover guard, you now have to pass their guard to get back to side control again.

*You can also add a mount transition into the mix too. The goal here is to start from side control and make your objective to advance to the mount while they're defending from their back. This leads nicely into the next drill.

Mount -

You start from the mount and your objective is to maintain mount control while they are aggressively defending from their back. You can add variables like submissions from the top as well. If your partner escapes the mount, you continue from whatever position you end up in.

Another option is to try and dismount and go from mount back to side control. This is a great way to practice your transitions into and then out of the mount without sacrificing position.

- Version #2 - If they reverse the position or there's an exchange of positions, you continue the action from wherever you end up.

Back -

The final main position is to work from back control. You can start with a seatbelt and both hooks / body triangle on. The goal is to maintain control without submitting them.

- Version #2 - If they reverse the position or there's an exchange of positions, you continue the action from wherever you end up.

- You can add more variables like: Having them start in turtle and you have to secure your seatbelt and then hooks. You can add submission attacks as well.

In this series of drills we covered the four main positions: Guard, Side Control, Mount and Back. You can also reverse the starting positions and you now start from the defensive side and they are the attacker. You can also start from secondary positions as well. For example: half guard, butterfly guard, De La Riva, open guard, deep half, single-leg X guard, etc.

Scenario based drilling -

The objective with this method is to put yourself in situations you will likely face in competition.

"**Bad day at the office**," escaping from bad positions -

You start from bad positions like: guard, side control, mount, back, etc. Your mission is to get yourself to a better position while staying calm and composed. You can add variables like having them intensify the pressure, attack with submissions, talk smack in your ear (just kidding), etc.

*You can add variables like starting from submissions. Just be mindful that you both agree that you will let your partner out of the move safely. With submissions you have to move slow and always allow ample time to escape or tap when needed.

"Down on points" -

The goal here is to simulate pressure and improve mental acuity. You start the drill by deciding that you're down by a certain number of points and you have only so much time left. For example: the score is 3-2 and you're losing and have 30-seconds left in the match. Someone signals the start of the time and you begin.

You can add variables like: starting from various positions (both good and bad). This could also include starting from within a submission. Like previously started, always be careful to not injure your training partner.

"Keeping the lead" and "Breaking the tie"-

With this drill you start with a one point lead and so much time left in the match. For example: it's 4-3 and you have 30 seconds left in your match. With the tie breaker drill you start with a score of 3-3 and you have 30 seconds to break the tie and win the match.

"Linking the chain" -

With this drill you connect moves together in sequences that fit into your game. For example: if you're a triangle choker, you might link the triangle from guard to an armbar, to a sweep, etc. You can add variables like having your partner create road blocks along the way. For example: when you go from the triangle to the armbar they might defend the arm and escape and you have to pick up the pieces.

"Getting outta hell" -

Your objective here is to start from your worst case scenario's like escaping submission attacks. For example: You have your partner start with you in an armbar and your job is to safely escape. Since you are starting from potentially dangerous, compromising positions you have to let your partner out before they need to tap. Since there's such a small space between tapping and an injury, only work from 30% speed and effort (or less). Agree ahead of time that you'll verbally say, "Tap, tap, tap!"

"Mastering the clock" -

Here you're focusing on time based scenarios. For example: you are down with a score of 5-4 and have 30-seconds left in the match. You can start from both good and bad positions and add whatever variables you like.

- Another option is to start with a one point lead and you have one minute to maintain the score without stalling. If you have a dominant position and are just trying to hold it without advancing, you can be warned and possibly penalized for stalling. It's important to be good at camouflaging your stalling tactics. The key here is to maintain position while looking like you're attacking. This can mean making grips on the collar and pulling and tugging. You want the referee to think you're trying to attack, when in fact you're riding the clock.

This can come into play when the have a score of 4-3 with 30 seconds left in the match and you're exhausted. You don't want to attack and then lose your position, and possibly lose the whole match. You have to trick the ref into thinking you are trying to get a submission, but really you're trying to survive and win.

If you want to be a successful competitor you have to learn to respect and master the clock. If your match is for five minutes, then you need to make sure you know exactly what five minutes of rolling under high intensity pressure feels like. It would be wonderful if you could win every match by submission, but it's just not the case. Some matches will go the time limit and you need to be adept at understanding the point system and time management of your match.

If you have a coach the day of the tournament they can help you by yelling the time left in the match and score to you. But this may not always be the case, so it's important for you to become a master at both the scoring system and time of your match.

Takedown drilling and preparation is another important component to consider. The challenge with starting from your feet is the risk of injury, particularly for over 40 athletes. I don't recommend full out, 100% grappling from your feet. The risk for injury is just too high. But you do have to prepare yourself for this aspect of the game. Unless you're a "guard-puller." There's often a little misguided "hate" thrown at guard players who don't do takedowns. The reality is that guard pulling is just an adaptation to the rules in BJJ competition. It's easier to just pull guard and most times the rules don't penalize it.

If you suck at takedowns, don't panic. You don't need a lot in your arsenal to be effective. I was personally never the greatest at takedowns, but I had one in particular that worked well for me. "Kosoto gake", known as the "minor outer hook" leg sweep. I have no idea where I learned it, but I was able to get it successfully in almost every competition match I've had. In fact, I've only pulled guard twice, ever. The reason it worked so well for me was partially my physical attributes of being long, tall and I have big feet. This allows this move to work well for me.

There is something to be said for finding 1-2 takedowns for your specific body style. Another reason Kosoto gake worked well for me was that it is a fairly low risk takedown. I'm 6'1" if I shot for a double leg, that might be really risky and put me in a worse position. However, if I was short and stocky that might be the perfect takedown for me. When you consider which takedowns to add to your toolbox, be sure they fit your physical attributes.

Here's a simple takedown formula where we match body styles to takedowns:

(These are a few examples of different takedowns. Don't limit yourself, dig into your own experience and arsenal of takedowns.)

- Tall, lanky and lean - Leg trips are going to be your best bet. Stay away from anything where you have to drop to your knees (i.e. double legs). For a taller person it is a long ways down to their knees and they can often anticipate the level change and defend the takedown. Whereas foot to foot sweeps are overall less risky. Longer legs in general can be more effective at entangling and controlling another persons legs. If you have long arms they can be effective for securing single leg takedowns and ankle picks.

- Preferred takedowns for a tall person - Kosoto gake, Uchi mata, Osoto gari, O Goshi (hip throw), Tani Otoshi (valley drop), Single leg, ankle picks, body fold, leg hook (inside and outside).

- Short and stocky - Double leg and single leg takedowns are excellent for those with a lower center of gravity. Drop Seoi Nagi and O Goshi (hip throw) are also excellent when you can get your hips underneath someone as a shorter person can do.

- Powerful upper body - Tai Otoshi (body drop), O Goshi (hip throw), Koshi Guruma (head lock throw), body fold takedown.

- Flexible and lean - Imanari roll, Yoko Tomoe Nage (side circular throw), fake guard pull to ankle pick. The fake guard pull works really well because as a smaller practitioner others will expect you to pull guard. Tani Otoshi (valley drop) is also excellent to feint a guard pull.

The takedowns listed here are just a few examples. Do some research and drilling to find the 1or 2 takedowns that you want to add to your game. Like I stated earlier, you don't need to have an entire toolbox of takedowns. Unless you have a strong background in Judo, Wrestling or Sambo - *then everyone else should keep it simple!*

Building a strong mental game will also be crucial to your tournament success. Start by managing your expectations. If this is your first tournament then embrace a growth mindset. Winning isn't just about getting a medal or championship belt. Every match, regardless of the outcome, is an opportunity for growth and expansion. Don't create additional anxiety by putting a lot of undue pressure on yourself. The goal is to enjoy the experience and learn something new along the way. Anything beyond those two will be considered added bonuses.

You also want to infuse a sense of resilience and adaptability into your training. When you compete you're definitely going to face challenges from both your competitors and your own nerves. There's no way to totally prepare for the unexpected in competition. It's best to be open to whatever happens, maintain focus and proactively adapt to the situation at hand.

This flexibility and adaptability can be cultivated in training by adding roadblocks during drilling. You can also make sure you're facing diverse, unpredictable situations during live rolling as well. The more "unforeseeable" events you can add, the better off you'll be later. Prepare and be open to all possibilities.

Visualization can be a powerful tool to add to your tournament prep. These powerful techniques can enhance performance, build confidence while easing your pre-competition jitters. Remember, words have power. The narrative you have playing on repeat in your mind will greatly impact your performance.

The following visualizations can help lay the groundwork for a positive outcome. When you practice mental imagery you want to do it in a quiet, comfortable space. Think of it like mediation. Be sure to relax your mind and body through your breath as you close your eyes and fabricate your mental movie. You can create and record your own visualizations or listen to the ones we've provided with this book.

Keep your visualization sessions to 5-10 minutes maximum. You can gradually increase your time as your focus improves. Keep your thoughts positive and use a first person perspective. See it through your own eyes as if you're doing it, not watching yourself do it. Engage all of your senses during your sessions. What does the room look like, smell like, sound like and feel like? Include as much emotion as possible. Are you elated, excited, happy, etc.? Like physical practice, the more you do it, the better you'll get at it.

"Facing challenges" - Imagine yourself in non-dominant positions, down on points, but you turn the tables and secure the victory. Don't be afraid to face your "worst case scenario's" now and overcome them in advance.

"Calm under fire" - Picture yourself in a tough position but you're calm, relaxed and in control. You don't panic but find a solution to the challenge.

"Flawless technique" - As you move through your 'go-to' moves you execute them with perfect technique and timing.

"Having fun" - See yourself smiling and having fun competing and meeting new people. Imagine yourself enjoying the thrill of competition and the camaraderie that accompanies it.

"Controlling the pace" - See yourself in a position of control, dictating the pace of the match. Even when challenges arise, you are able to control the outcome with confidence and resilience.

"Loose and flexible" - Your body feels great and you can move pain-free and with ease and mobility. You see yourself easily slipping in and out of moves.

"Recovering from errors" - Picture yourself making a mistake but immediately recovering and readjusting your game plan. Imagine you're calm and relaxed.

In the same way you train your body, visualization trains your mind to positively react to challenging scenarios. By repeating these sessions you build familiarity around what would otherwise be uncomfortable situations. By facing these obstacles in the present moment you pre-pave a path of successful responses and decision-making under pressure. The more consistent you are at practicing within the safety of your mind, the stronger the neural pathways, and better prepared you'll be when it happens in competition. Visualization is a powerful tool that can help you become a better competitor and stronger person in general.

Positive affirmations can also help to shift your mindset, making you less anxious about your upcoming competition. These short, powerful statements can help reset our thinking and subsequently influence our behaviors and habits. The general concept is to redirect negative thought patterns with positive, affirming statements. In this section we share positive affirmations for competition. These should be repeated often, like a song playing relentlessly in your head.

"My age is my advantage"

"I am strong, confident and prepared"

"I am flexible and prepared for every possibility"

"I am confident in my preparation"

"I am calm and focused under pressure"

"I trust in my strategy"

"I believe in my Jiu-Jitsu!"

"Win or lose, I'm here for the lessons"

"My age brings wisdom"

"I am calm and in control of my emotions"

"Every roll brings me closer to my goal!"

"I am flexible and adaptable"

"I thrive under pressure"

"I welcome the rush!"

"I move with ease"

"Competing is the accomplishment!"

"I trust in my technique"

"I respect my opponents, but I am not intimidated by them"

"I'm ready for what's next"

"It feels so good when I did it and it's done!"

You can also create your own list of affirmations that align with your goals and objectives. Be specific and make it personal!

Mission:

Preparation is not just about physical readiness but also about mental and logistical planning. Comprehensive preparation increases confidence and performance.

Introduce more cognitive and psychological prep work into the pre-tournament routines.

Start a tournament preparation checklist that includes mental conditioning, diet adjustments, and logistical planning starting one month before the event.

Survival Expert:
VLADISLAV (Vlad) KOULIKOV

BJJ Black Belt First degree under Professor Rafael "Formiga" Barbosa, Sambo Master Of Sport, Judo Sandan, Sambo coach Sfrgei Vorotyagin

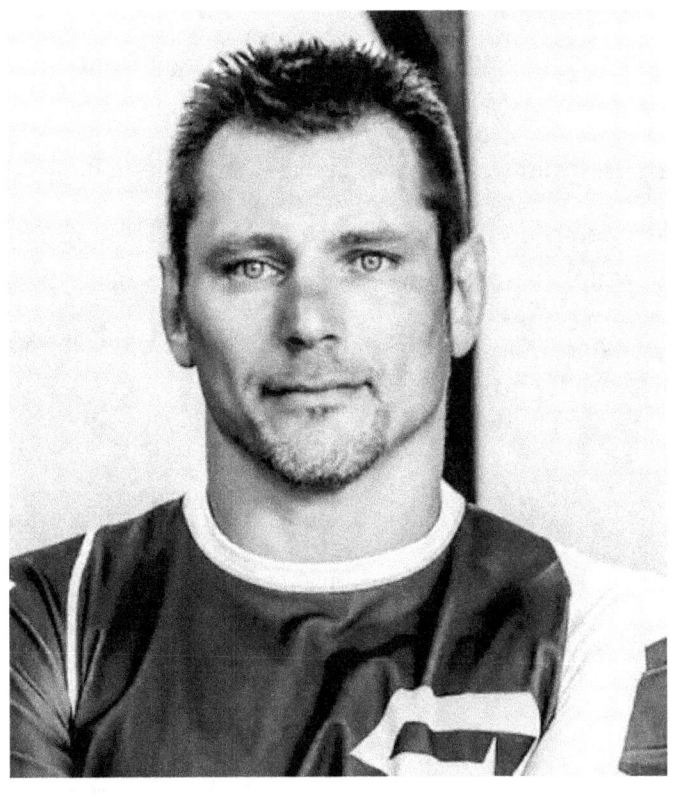

Intel:

Vlad is a world champion competitor; placing three times in the USA Open and represented team USA in combat SAMBO in the World Championship in 2008. Placed and won multiple NAGA and Grapplers Quest tournaments and was awarded the most technical fighter in the very first Grapplers Quest competition winning all his matches by submissions. He has been training in the Russian martial art of Sambo from a very young age in Moscow. Since moving to the USA, he has trained and competed in submission grappling and wrestling.

From the Source:

As you might know I'm not a pure Jiujitero. I enjoy grappling in all its forms, shapes and rule sets.

Once you have fundamental knowledge of principles you can start educating yourself.

Rolling exposes your weaknesses and that's what you should work on.

As an older competitor I urge you to NOT obsess about aging. There is grace and wisdom in that. However one can't be oblivious to the changes.

I realized after a couple serious injuries that I'm not bulletproof and it's okay to reject rolls or cherry pick them.

Another thing -

I realize how much good training habits affect your overall performance.

I started to treat my training time more economically -

I can't afford wasting time doing unneeded stuff.

Don't neglect the recovery process!

Good sleep, proper eating habits, self care (massage, chiropractic adjustment, hot / cold exposure) became as important as rolling and drilling.

I stopped working out heavily, I simply don't need that anymore.

Time spent free moving on the mat, drilling or rolling an extra round is way better spent.

Stage III: Analyzing Performance

In this section we will discuss tips and strategies for having a successful tournament day! These lessons all come from a lifetime of competing and coaching others. Many of which I and others had to learn the "hard way."

The night's sleep before your big day is crucial. You don't want to spend it tossing and turning only to wake up after an hour's hard sleep. You're now expected to go and compete on a zero night's rest? That's not a good idea! If you're planning on traveling and sleeping in a hotel you may need to make adjustments. Try to recreate your normal home sleeping environment. Whatever pillows you normally use, bring them along on the trip. If you use a body pillow, bring it too. If you have a favorite blanket or little sleeping buddy, bring them all. I jest... but seriously, the objective is for it to feel like a normal nights sleep.

What to pack for your tournament:

Clothing:

- Change of clothing for after competing.

- Flip flops for the tournament. This is very important for rest room trips. If a competitor is spotted using a restroom in bare feet they can be disqualified.

This is unsanitary and potentially dangerous due to possible skin infections.

- Hoodie to wear at the tournament over your rash guard / gi. This will keep you warm and comfortable. A zip up hoodie is best as it's easier to get on and off.
- Sleep wear
- Sneakers
- Tournament towel for wiping sweat. A second towel for after the competition. This will be used for cleaning off and drying yourself before leaving the event.
- Travel clothes (comfortable for a car ride) and a change of clothing for your stay. Also have a few clean outfits for post competition. A sweat suit for after competing and something comfortable for the ride home.

Toiletries:

- Body wash and shampoo
- Deodorant / body spray
- Mints / gum
- Shaving kit
- Tooth brush, tooth paste, mouth wash. Have mouth wash or mints available for a quick clean and rinse before competing.

*Have them available post-competition for a quick cleaning before hitting the road.

Post-comp skin care - It's extremely important to leave the tournament with clean skin. You don't want to bring anything nasty home for your teammates or family.

- More than likely you won't be able to shower after you compete. Also chances are you will be checked out of your hotel too. Therefore you have to clean yourself properly before a long ride home. Do not get into your car with someone else's nasty dried sweat on your body.

- Wash all of your exposed skin with antimicrobial soap. Especially your exposed limbs, hands, feet, face and neck. Use your clean towel to dry off. Change into an entire set of clean, dry clothes. (Including under garments) Don't wear the sweaty, wet rash guard home! Also don't take off the rash guard and throw on the new tournament tee shirt you bought. Clean yourself first, then put on your shiny new shirt!

- You can also use full body, disposable body wipes. These are a good back up plan if there's no where to properly wash your body. Antiseptic skin sprays also work well when you're in a pinch to disinfect any exposed skin.

Health and wellness:

Pain relief body spray. ("Bio freeze") These work well on sore, tender areas. You can use it before or after the competition for pain relief. (No greasy, smelly skin creams during competition)

Band-aids

Athletic tape for fingers or joints

Ibuprofen

Bag of epsom salts for a hot bath

Container or hand sanitizer

Nutrition and hydration:

Reusable water bottle with plenty of water. (A gallon bottle is a safe bet so you have plenty on hand).

Fruit / veggie snacks: Bananas, oranges, apples, grapes, pineapple, carrots, celery (Pick a few that you like)

Protein bars

Hydration / electrolyte packets

Pre-made sandwiches and snack items

Over-pack on food, you'll thank me later. It's best to go overboard on food and snacks. You can pack everything in a big cooler.

Competition gear:

Be sure to review the gi, belt and rash guard requirements ahead of the competition day.

Gi and belt (bring an extra gi)

Rash guard, spats (tights), shorts, under garments for competing.

Compression sleeves, if any (knees, ankles, etc.)

Athletic tape

Mouth piece (check rules)

Extra pair of flip flops

Watch or timer

*Make sure all of your gear is free from tears and rips.

Other essentials:

ID / passport (if needed)

Cash and credit cards

Phone and charger

Headphones and charger

Entertainment: Book, iPad, music, ear phones, etc.

Music playlist for the competition

Confirmation of tournament registration

Directions and address of the venue

Somewhere to store your valuables while competing ("Master Lock" sells a portable small lock box that can be cable locked to a bag or seat - available on Amazon for under $25)

It is imperative that you get a good nights sleep before competing. Sometimes trying to get to sleep can cause even more anxiety and keep you awake even longer. The objective is to create the best possible conditions for rest. If you're traveling try to find a hotel / motel with a pool and preferably hot tub. The night before the tournament you can swim and soak after a good meal. I always followed my swim with a nice long evening walk. If there's no pool then soak in your room bath tub. Stop into a local store (or pack ahead of time) epsom salts for your hot soak. They will relax and calm your muscles before sleep.

A evening walk will also calm your nerves and let you release any additional nervous energy you may be harboring. You can follow this up with a nice stretch and meditation before you sleep. Like we mentioned earlier in this section, if you're traveling bring all of your favorite pillows and comfort items to ensure a restful nights sleep.

You may also consider bringing some familiar music or a favorite book to help lull you to sleep. The goal is to replicate your home sleeping arrangements while in a hotel. Ear plugs are also great to have on hand for any loud hotel guests. Make sure you set your alarm for a hardy breakfast meal. You need to make sure you start the day with a full stomach even if you are nervous and don't feel like eating. Your body will need the energy from food to fuel your big day. Aim for something robust and nutritious. A bowl of oatmeal, a protein smoothie, eggs, fruit, etc. can all be a good start to your day. Even after you eat, plan on snacking and hydrating throughout the day. It's imperative that you keep yourself fueled and ready.

Don't show up when the doors open! There's no rush to get there. You'll just stir up nervous energy and exhaust yourself mentally and physically. If you have a scheduled time for your match, arrive an hour or two beforehand. You just need enough time to change and warm up. If you have to arrive early to support fellow teammates or family members, don't get changed into your competition gear. You don't want to be tempted to stretch and warm up all day. Conserve your energy. Try to chill out as much as possible when you're spectating. Don't burn a lot of energy by yelling, cheering and coaching. Those constant highs will deplete your gas tank. Don't blow all of your energy on everyone else's match. Protect your spark!

You'll want to keep your energy levels high by eating nutritious snacks and hydrating throughout the day. The combination of food, fluids and nervousness may keep you going to the restrooms. Don't let that sway you from eating and consuming water.

- What to do if you don't have a coach. First off, prepare ahead of time. If you know that you don't have a coach or teammate then you might have to fly solo. If you have a coach that's great. You'll want to confirm that they can be at your mat at the designated time you're competing.

There's three types of coaches at a tournament:

1. Professor or coach

2. Teammate

3. Alone or just a time keeper

The professor or coach is someone who knows your game and can be an asset to you while competing. This is the ideal situation. Your regular coach has three important roles. 1 - Announce the time and score for you 2 - Keep you focused and motivated during your match 3 - Be your second set of eyes, coach you on specific moves and help you predict and adapt to the changing circumstances.

Your teammate, depending on their level, will be able to do everything a coach can do. The difference (which can be vast) is the level of experience they can provide. Although a purple belt who has competed multiple times might be an excellent coach. Whereas an inexperienced white or blue belt may be more limited in their coaching ability.

If you're alone don't panic! I've competed many, many times without a coach or time keeper. If you are flying solo that just means you need to be hyper focused during your match.

You can't ever lose track of these three critical elements:

1. Where am I? And where am I going? (position-wise)

2. What is the score of the match?

3. How much time is left?

There's obviously much more going on during a tournament match. But if you're alone, it's best to keep the playbook simple. Don't try to juggle too many plates at once. I would even recommend constantly checking in with yourself during the match. Keep asking yourself the three critical elements. This will keep you focused and grounded in the present moment.

For example, let's say you're on your back. You start by asking, "Where am I?" Followed by the question, "Where am I going? You answer by mentally saying, "He's in my half guard and I want to sweep him." That answers where are you and where are you going. You start by evaluating your position. You then ask, what is the score of the match and how much time is left? This also help you formulate your plan. The score might be 4-2 and you're winning with 30 - seconds left. In that scenario you may want to just hold onto the lead and go for the win.

It's not easy to build a strategy on the fly without a second set of eyes and experience. I call the voice in my head "J.A.R.V.I.S." like the voice that Iron Man hears that guides him during his adventures. In the Marvel Universe J.A.R.V.I.S stands for "Just A Rather Very Intelligent System." It's an artificial intelligence system that speaks to Tony Stark when he's in his suit. Jarvis manages the technology of his suit and provides critical intelligence when he's in combat situations. So like Tony Stark, you have to use the technology of your conscious mind to keep yourself alert and fully engaged in your match. You want to avoid going into "fight or flight" and completely blanking out. To keep yourself fully present always find your way back to the "three critical elements."

You can practice this during drilling. At different intervals during grappling matches in training check in with your inner-Jarvis and ask your three questions. You can even set a timer or have a partner verbally say, "Three!" When they give you the "three" signal, your job is to announce your three questions. For example: You say, 1. "Guard and trying to set up a sweep," 2. "The score is 5-2," 3. "There's 3 minutes left in the round"

Once again, you state where you are and where you're going, the score of the match and the time remaining.

*If possible, video record your matches. This will come in handy later when you can evaluate your performance.

The most important piece of advice surrounding tournaments is to have fun! Seriously enjoy the experience. Don't make it some huge, monumental, overwhelming event. Try to enjoy every aspect it. Don't get lost in the thirst to win. Yes, you want to get on the medal stand. But don't let the ambition to win overshadow the opportunity for inner growth. Regardless of how the experience turns out, there's always a possibility for a bigger lesson. Be open and looking for that possibility.

Mission:

Execution on competition day depends heavily on the preceding preparations. The ability to stay calm and adapt strategies on the fly is crucial.

Focus more on adaptive strategies during the competition to handle unexpected challenges or changes in brackets.

Engage in simulation drills that introduce unexpected changes or challenges, mimicking potential competition day surprises.

Stage IV: Beyond the Score

You did it! Regardless of whether it was your first or one hundredth tournament, you deserve the recognition. Even if it didn't turn out the way you would have liked. Even if you got choked out in the first ten seconds, you deserve the acknowledgment. It takes guts for anyone to compete in a combat sport like BJJ. It also takes a special breed of human to do it after 40 years old! That deserves to be validated.

Your first step after a tournament is give your body the rest and recovery it needs and deserves. A soak in an epsom salt bath can be a perfect way to reduce soreness and inflammation while spending some time in reflection. You can use this time to replay the entire experience like you're watching a mental movie. Look for the highlights and areas of improvement. Don't beat the hell out of yourself in regret. Note where you can make improvements and get ready to implement them in training.

- If you have video of your matches, schedule a private lesson with your professor or coach to review your performance. This is a vital opportunity to improve, so don't disregard it. Most importantly, don't be embarrassed by your performance. It takes guts to compete!

You have to anticipate that you will be extremely sore after completing. You can pre-schedule a massage for 2-3 days after you compete. Don't schedule it for the day after as you will still be tender from competing and probably won't feel like a massage. It's better to wait a day or two after your body is somewhat recovered. If you didn't medal at your first tournament, don't despair, as most people don't. Apply the lessons you've gained and get right back on the horse! Look for the next tournament and get signed up now.

Mission:

First off, let me start by saying that not everyone will want to, nor should they compete in grappling tournaments. Only you and your professor will know this for sure. But even if you decide to never compete, you will come across students and teammates who will want to. Regardless of what your feelings are about competition, it's not fair to hold someone else back from their pursuits. So my point is that learning and embracing this knowledge for yourself and others is invaluable. For non-competitors, you can also use the drills and strategies here to improve your in-class grappling performance. I'm not saying to treat open mat like a tournament. But rather use this knowledge to take your grappling to the next level!

Or perhaps if you've never competed before, then maybe it's time to plan your "ninja-recon mission." The goal is to go and watch a tournament in person. This experience will help you form a better opinion on whether you should pursue this endeavor. If you plan on competing or already compete, then it's time to take it to level eleven. One of the best pieces of tournament advice came from my black belt wife. She once told me, "to act and train like a professional!" This simple phrase was game changing for me. Her point was that I should think, eat, breathe, sleep, train and recover like a professional athlete. You might be competing in a local tournament, but think of the edge you would have by approaching it in this manner?

To be in your best form requires a multi-faceted approach. This includes your diet, both physical and mental, as well as how you approach training and recovery, all of which will directly affect your performance on the day of the event. You can leave no stone unturned. By embracing every aspect of this book, you'll be on the path to success both in competition and in life.

Debriefing Assessment:

Reflect on your preparation for the competition, considering both your physical readiness and mental strategies. Did your training regimen adequately prepare you for the intensity of the competition? Evaluate your performance against your personal expectations and the goals you set.

Identify specific areas where adjustments are needed. For instance, if stamina was an issue, consider integrating more cardiovascular training into your routine. If technique execution faltered under pressure, plan targeted drills to enhance muscle memory and response time under stress.

Gather feedback from coaches, peers, and your own observations to inform future strategies. Was there a common theme in the feedback regarding your defensive tactics or aggression levels? Use this information to refine your approach.

If, you're still interested in competing, set concrete goals for your next competition. These might include technical improvements, mental conditioning, or recovery strategies. Establish a timeline for achieving these goals to maintain focus and momentum in your training.

PART III:
OFF THE MATS -
INTEGRATING BJJ INTO LIFE

Operations:

3.0

Tailored focus is placed on advanced techniques to maintain muscle mass, manage injuries, and integrate strategic recovery. It's about enhancing flexibility and ensuring ongoing vitality in your BJJ.

Scan the QR code for in-depth analysis
and expert commentary.

https://www.youtube.com/playlist?list=PLwb5iQup993
_ZEmE-EZlhlLg4GRnwBVQ8

Long Term Injuries

To mend the vessel, you must first fortify the spirit. Jiu-Jitsu serves as a gateway to mastering the flow of our internal energies. Embrace your practice of martial arts not as exercises but as rituals—like a ceremony of healing and empowerment. We have the capacity to reshape our perception of pain, turning it from a hindrance into a source of strength. This isn't just about endurance but rewriting the narratives that bind us.

- Consider using a different way to speak to yourself. Make your own language to alter pain perception, enhance motivation, and reinforce the mind-body connection. Each time you spar you can reframe challenges as opportunities, transforming the dojo into a crucible where the true steel of our spirit is forged.

Remember—the path of the warrior is eternally unfolding. Embrace it all.

Research Yourself: Become the expert on your own body. Understanding the root of your injury helps in adapting your training and managing your recovery process effectively.

Adjust Intensity and Volume: Reduce and modify your game accordingly to accommodate your body's healing process. Shift your focus to precision rather than strength or endurance.

Technique Over Sparring: Prioritize drilling and technique work over live sparring to minimize risk of aggravating your injury.

Alternative Exercises: Incorporate exercises that strengthen muscles around the injured area without putting direct stress on it. For example, if you have a knee injury, focus on upper body and core strength.

Reinforcement and Prevention

Strengthening and Conditioning: Regular strength and conditioning tailored to BJJ can help prevent injuries by strengthening the muscles, joints, and ligaments used in the sport.

Flexibility and Mobility: Incorporate flexibility and mobility work into your routine to reduce the risk of injuries and aid in recovery.

Protective Gear: Use appropriate protective gear, such as knee braces or ear guards, to protect vulnerable areas during training.

Adapt Your Lifestyle

Nutrition: Proper nutrition supports injury recovery. Focus on a balanced diet rich in vitamins, minerals, and proteins to aid in the healing process.

Rest and Recovery: Adequate rest is crucial. Ensure you're getting enough sleep and consider incorporating active recovery days to promote healing.

Mindset: Adopt a positive and patient mindset. Understand that recovery takes time and rushing the process can lead to further injury

Listen to Your Body

Pain as a Guide: Use pain as a guide for your training intensity. If something hurts, avoid it or find a way to modify the movement.

Monitor and Adapt: Regularly assess your pain and injury status. Be prepared to adapt your training based on your body's feedback.

Professional Guidance for Long-Term Management

Physical Therapy: Engage in physical therapy specifically designed for your injury and BJJ. A physical therapist can provide exercises and routines to strengthen the injured area and prevent future injuries.

Regular Check-Ups: Regular medical check-ups can help monitor your injury and recovery process, allowing for adjustments in your training regimen as needed.

Community Support

Share Experiences: Engage with the BJJ community, especially with practitioners who have gone through similar experiences. Sharing tips and advice can be incredibly beneficial.

Coach Communication: Maintain open communication with your coach and professors about your injury and limitations. A knowledgeable coach can help modify your training while keeping your skills sharp.

Incorporating these tips into your training regimen can help you manage and recover from injuries while continuing to practice BJJ. Remember, the goal is longevity in the sport, and taking care of your body is paramount to achieving this.

Mission:

Modifications in training routines are crucial for practitioners dealing with chronic pain, allowing them to train effectively without exacerbating conditions.

Include more alternative training methods like aqua training or yoga that are easier on the joints.

Weekly sessions focused on non-impact BJJ techniques and complementary physical activities that support long-term joint health.

Everything Flexibility to Roll With It

Stretching for an after 40 BJJ practice is imperative for preventing injuries. When we discuss the importance of off the mats training we cannot emphasize enough the importance of an ongoing flexibility program.

When it comes to stretching most people fall into one of three categories.

1. "Feel like I've never been flexible, and never will"

2. "I'm moderately flexible, but with limitations"

3. "I have been fairly flexible my whole life, but it's becoming more difficult to maintain as I age"

The advantage of adding flexibility is twofold. Firstly, it will keep you safer during training and aid in a faster recovery. Secondly, you'll have more tools at your disposal when you're rolling. You don't need to be able to stick your legs behind your neck, but having a moderate level of flexibility is important. One of the greatest benefits of stretching for over 40 athletes is the increased range of motion in their joints. You've heard the saying, "If it doesn't bend it will break." You don't want to be on the breaking end of a wildly executed "bend."

When you're drilling with partners you want to ensure that you have a good range of motion and never allow them to "squeeze" submissions when they're drilling joint locks. The repeated locking out of the joints against a fulcrum can cause additional, unnecessary wear and tear. Injuries like tendonitis are often the cause of over extending joint locks. Developing a good range of motion allows you to move fluidly with the technique, not against it. Keeping your joints relaxed and calm during drilling will help. Good communication is also key. Always have your tapping hand at the ready and be extra prepared for a verbal, "Tap, tap, tap!"

When I train joint locks I always tell my partners to go at 20-30% speed, this gives me ample time to protect my joints. It also allows for a slow steady stream of pressure that is safer on the joints as we age. To improve your flexibility you have to stretch consistently. Of course results will vary from individual to individual. Natural flexibility can differ based on genetics, muscle length, age, ligaments, body composition, etc. Many factors come into play. But with some dedicated work everyone can improve their results. For us over 40 players we are going to keep this simple and easy as stretching protocols can get unnecessarily complicated. For your purposes as a BJJ practitioner we'll keep it as straight forward as possible.

The two primary methods for flexibility are static and dynamic stretching. Generally speaking static stretching is where you hold a stretch in place for 15-30 seconds. Experts say this method can help lengthen the muscle over time and also aid in recovery. It may reduce muscle soreness and aid in the removal of lactic acid.

Dynamic stretching on the other hand mixes movement with flexibility. For BJJ purposes I prefer dynamic stretching (with a little mix of static) as it closely mimics the fluidity of grappling. Have you ever heard BJJ being referred to as "murder yoga" because of the compromising positions we put each other in? The practice of Jiu-Jitsu is a constant interplay of movement, balance, and leverage.

Because BJJ is a technique based martial art that focuses heavily on efficiency in action, dynamic stretching can be very effective. The more fluid and technical the movements are the less effort is needed. Dynamic stretching aligns perfectly with this concept. It can also serve as an excellent precursor to live grappling. Think of it as a warm up that prepares your body for the twisting, torquing, pretzel-like positions of grappling.

Tips for starting a consistent flexibility program:

Create a stretching area - You don't need a huge matted area. A yoga mat that's tucked behind your couch or under your bed works great.

Keep it simple and start slow - Remember, "slow and steady always wins the race." You don't need to stretch for hours on end every day. Start simple with a 10-15 minute routine. Set a timer for ten minutes then see how you feel after the initial session. You can always go a little longer, but don't overdue it! As you progress you can utilize your Pomodoro method for stretching. Set your timer for 25 minutes of uninterrupted stretching with a five minute break. Then reevaluate if you want to go longer.

Set and setting - It can be far more enjoyable when you have your headphones and some good music playing when you stretch. Ambient music can also be playing in the background if you want to meditate while you move your body. This type of music can have a calming and grounding effect. I'm a big classic hard rock kind of guy, but for stretching I keep it pretty chilled out.

Warm up - Start with slow controlled movements that give your body time to adapt. Adding controlled, rhythmic breathing can help keep you stay relaxed and calm allowing for better range of motion. Try to exhale on the most difficult portion of the stretch. This is generally as you are bending forward. A good rule of thumb is, exhale when your head is moving towards your legs. You should inhale as your head moves away from your legs (when your chest expanding, this equals an exhalation).

Jiu-Jitsu specific movements - You want your movements to mimic the way you play BJJ. If you like triangles and omoplata's then add those movements to your routine. Since BJJ is a full body martial art, you want to engage your whole being. Be sure to give extra attention to your neck, spine, back and hips and legs as these are all used constantly during grappling.

Document your routines in your BJJ notebook - When you write it down you'll feel more accountable to completing the objective. Plus there's a dopamine hit and a sense of accomplishment from following through on your goals. Dopamine is part of your brain's reward system. Experts say that the bigger the task completed, the bigger the hit!

Mission:

This operation is vital because it will set the tone for your time on the mat. Remember, if your recovery time is left unattended to, your body will surely let you know! With this mission we must first address how many days per week you will spend actively training in Jiu-Jitsu. As discussed earlier, my recommendation is 2-3 times per week for beginners (white belts), 3-4 for blue belts and higher. Sure we would all love to train more but we need balance our on the mat time with stretching, recovery, family, work and life! I would love to eat pizza every day but I realize that's not sustainable. You might respond with, "of course not, pizza isn't healthy!" Neither is too much Jiu-Jitsu. By approaching your BJJ in a healthy, balanced manner we create true longevity. Once you have scheduled your BJJ and weight training, you then have to choose your recovery days and plan.

As we discussed, flexibility serves as a great form of recovery and added BJJ skill set. The more flexible you are, the more you can do on the mats. If you're about as bendable as a rusty tin man, don't despair. There's hope for you too, but YOU have to take action! Now get on the floor and stretch, *it's really that simple.*

Survival Expert: BONG ABAD / GAWAKOTO

age 49, BJJ black belt under Saulo Ribeiro

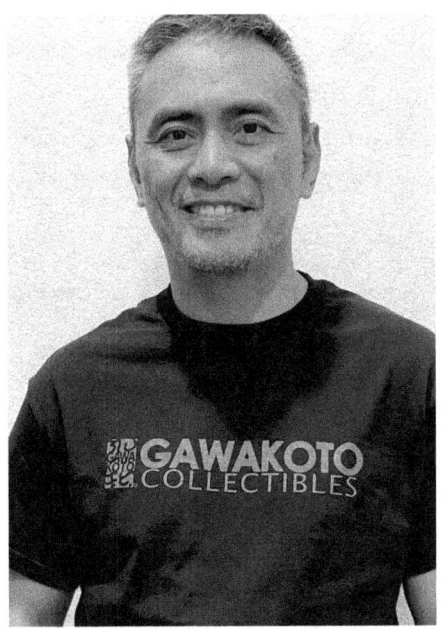

Intel:

I became friends with Bong Abad aka "Gawakoto" through his amazing designs. I was gifted one of his tee shirts by a student and fell in love with his work. I have always been a fan of comic book art my entire life. Bong's work was very reminiscent of the comic-style art work I admired as a teenager.

When I learned that Bong was also a Jiu-Jitsu junkie, I became an even bigger fan. Over the past few years I have watched him interact with members on the BJJAfter40 Facebook group. He is always kind, supportive and offers invaluable advice for smaller over 40 athletes.

Straight from the Source:

I'm Bong Abad aka Gawakoto (pseudonym I've used since the launch of my brand). I was born and raised in the Philippines and currently residing in San Diego. I am a new black belt under Ribeiro Jiu-Jitsu. I started training BJJ in the UK under Nic Gregoriades' Jiu-Jitsu Brotherhood. I moved to the US and trained at the, now defunct, University of Jiu-Jitsu, home gym of Saulo & Xande Ribeiro. Right now, I am training under Julio Villanueva, (currently) under the Ribeiro banner. I've been training Jiu-Jitsu now for 10 1/2 yrs, and received my black belt in 2021.

I only competed when I was a blue belt. I didn't enjoy the experience. Competition just didn't appeal to me. My goal in Jiu-Jitsu is mainly for self-defense and fitness. However, since I got my black belt, I've been enjoying teaching. Which I intend to do more and be better at.

I choose my partners 'wisely.' **It's important that you are aware of how your teammates roll, and that you are attuned to their energy / vibes.** Some people are just 'hard rollers' no matter what the situation is. These are the ones who are always in "competition mode" or just new to the sport. They will use their strength at their disposal. These are the people you need to avoid, especially when you are tired. When you can't avoid it (being paired by the instructor or something, or just up for the challenge that day), play your defensive game - practice your frames, hip escape / switch etc. play not be 'tapped' rather than going on the offensive. Most likely, they will match that energy, and if they are inexperienced the likelihood of injury is high.

- Be aware of your own body. And when something doesn't feel right, it's mostly like that there is a potential for injury. It is wise to tap at this point. You don't want to be in a point of no return. Tap early.

BJJ has helped me develop my confidence. As a kid, I've always been shy. As I've progressed with the sport, I've found myself able to express myself more, either verbally or artistically. It is through Jiu-Jitsu that I managed to build my brand 'Gawakoto'. From making gi's to toys, my artistic output has always been influenced partly by Jiu-Jitsu; the other being, comics.

Jiu-Jitsu is keeping me healthy. So, I train at least one time a week. Despite family & work schedule, **I always try to make time to train**. Whether that be drilling sessions or sparring.

I eat fairly healthily keeping my weight on check most of the time. Keeping my food sources varied and not strictly on a specified diet.

I was a 'weakling' as a kid. Never the athletic type. I am just a year shy of being 50 and this is the fittest I've ever been. I'm not on any medications or have any major illness. And despite doing Jiu-Jitsu up to now, never had surgery of any kind. However, recently developed carpal tunnel syndrome on my hands. But that is more from sculpting and drawing, I think. Aggressive gripping in Jiu-Jitsu seems to contribute as well.

I like the challenges that Jiu-Jitsu imposes despite my diminishing physical attributes due to advancing age. Learning new techniques keeps my body and mind fresh and hungry for more.

Train smart. Listen to your body.

Keeping Energy Levels Up

In the pursuit of Jiu-Jitsu excellence, energy management is as critical as technique. For the mature athlete, maintaining high energy levels isn't just about physical conditioning; it's a holistic endeavor that encompasses diet, sleep, and mental well-being.

Nutritional Tactics

Energy sustenance starts with what you fuel your body with. Incorporate a balanced diet rich in complex carbohydrates, lean proteins, and healthy fats. Carbohydrates are the fuel that powers your training sessions, proteins repair and build muscle tissues, and fats support cellular function. Don't overlook hydration—water is crucial for maintaining energy as it aids in nutrient transportation and body temperature regulation.

Sleep Strategies

Recovery is your secret weapon. Quality sleep is non-negotiable, as it allows for both physical and mental recovery. Aim for 7-9 hours of sleep per night, ensuring that you enter deep sleep cycles crucial for m'uscle repair and cognitive function. Consider developing a pre-sleep routine that might include meditation or reading, aiding in the transition to restful slumber.

Mental Resilience

Mental fatigue can drain energy levels faster than physical exertion. Develop mental resilience through meditation, mindfulness, and cognitive exercises like visualization. Visualizing successful techniques and matches can boost confidence and conserve energy spent on anxiety and stress.

Mission:

Evaluate and adjust your diet for a week, focusing on nutrient-rich foods that enhance energy.

Set a strict sleep schedule and stick to it, utilizing relaxation techniques to improve sleep quality.

Spend 15 minutes daily on mental training, such as meditation or visualization, to enhance focus and reduce energy waste.

Track and optimize your diet for two weeks, focusing on balancing macronutrients and incorporating energy-boosting foods.

Monitor your hydration daily, setting reminders to drink water, especially before and after training.

Maintaining Muscle Mass and Gaining Strength

As Jiu-Jitsu practitioners age, maintaining muscle mass and strength becomes a formidable challenge. The mastery of this art demands not just skill but also physical capability, which can be sustained through targeted training and dietary strategies.

Strength Training - Incorporate strength training into your routine at least twice a week. Focus on compound movements such as squats, deadlifts, and bench presses, which recruit multiple muscle groups, promoting hormone balance and muscle growth. Use resistance training to complement BJJ, enhancing both strength and endurance.

Protein Intake - Protein is essential for muscle repair and growth. Increase your protein intake to match your training demands, aiming for 1.2 to 2.0 grams of protein per kilogram of body weight daily. Spread your protein consumption throughout the day to maximize absorption and muscle protein synthesis.

Recovery Techniques - Effective recovery accelerates muscle repair and growth. Incorporate active recovery sessions, such as light swimming or yoga, which stimulate blood flow and help reduce soreness. Utilize massage and stretching to maintain muscle elasticity and performance.

Mission:

Implement a structured strength training program tailored to your BJJ needs.

Adjust your daily diet to include adequate protein from diverse sources.

Dedicate time for active recovery weekly, focusing on techniques that enhance muscle recovery and growth.

Conditioning exercises not only help maintain muscle mass but also improve your cardiovascular health, which is vital for long training sessions. Incorporate activities like cycling, rowing, or brisk walking into your routine at least three times a week.

Set a three-month goal for strength training, including specific exercises tailored to enhancing your BJJ performance.

Plan meals weekly to ensure a high protein intake every day, considering both natural and supplementary sources.

Commit to a regular conditioning schedule, gradually increasing intensity to challenge your body and build endurance.

Debriefing Assessment:

These chapters reaffirm the non-negotiables in BJJ—recognizing early signs of injury and responding with appropriate interventions. It underlines the importance of prehab routines over mere rehab, promoting a preventive rather than reactive approach to physical health.

The discussions around flexibility are not confined to physicality but extend to the adaptability of training routines and life roles as one ages. This serves not only as a means to enhance performance but also as a strategy to minimize injuries.

At the core of sustaining practice over decades is the management of energy and the strategic development of strength. These chapters offer innovative ways to integrate strength training that complements BJJ, ensuring that muscle mass and energy levels support rather than hinder growth in the art.

Jiu-Jitsu is as much about fighting against opponents on the mat as it is about combating the internal and external limitations imposed by time. It champions a philosophy of continuous adaptation and learning, which is essential not just for survival but for thriving in the lifelong practice of Brazilian Jiu-Jitsu.

Operations:

<u>Life</u>

Discussions on balancing BJJ with life's responsibilities, health and wellness, and incorporating mindfulness and mental health practices.

Scan the QR code for insights into life lessons learned through
Brazilian Jiu-Jitsu.

https://www.youtube.com/playlist?list=PLwb5iQup9939
Op4Gi00qxmDKgpk86l8FV

Balancing BJJ, Family and Work

Finding a happy medium between your personal life, your professional life, and your BJJ training takes effort, but it's attainable with the right approach. The last thing we want is for their to be resentment with our loved ones towards our Jiu-Jitsu training. We all have different responsibilities that fill our lives. Whether we have young (or grown kids), dogs, horses, cars, we all face lifestyle scheduling challenges. In this section we will share tips on creating the perfect equilibrium of BJJ and life. I personally think of myself as a "Martial Artist" first and foremost. There's no reality where Jiu-Jitsu doesn't fit into my life. Yes, I know it's my career and you may be a part time practitioner. But it hasn't always been this way for me too.

I have had to maintain my own sense of balance. It's a juggling act. But like any good performer, when I drop the balls, I pick them up and start again. It takes skill to strike the perfect balance.

Start by deciding what's achievable. In order to develop balance you must set goals that are attainable. You don't (and shouldn't) train 5 or 6 days per week. It's not realistic or sustainable. As a 40-plus practitioner you want to balance weight training with BJJ training. Three days of BJJ training with 2-4 days of weight lifting is perfect for most people. You will get what you need from the mats while still building your strength and armor.

Remember that consistency is more valuable than intensity in the long term, especially when you prioritize quality over quantity. If you trained Jiu-Jitsu three days per week, you would open up more time for family and work responsibilities. Your weight training can easily be done at home or at the gym during off times. This will allow you more flexibility in your schedule.

Whenever possible schedule your days and weeks in advance, setting aside time each day for BJJ, your family, and your job. It's important to plan downtime for other hobbies, social events, and of course recuperation.

Maintaining a healthy work-life balance requires constant and open dialogue with loved ones and coworkers. Make sure your family and friends know how beneficial BJJ is to your health and mental well being. In addition, if you need to adjust your working hours to accommodate training, talk to your boss about it. When you return from BJJ practice share how you feel with your loved ones. This is a great way to express appreciation for everyone allowing you the space and time to train. You might say something like, *"I feel so great from BJJ class, thank you for being flexible so that I can train."* Then through your actions extend that gratitude by sharing your joy with your family. You don't want to come home from BJJ in a worse mood!

Making your training a family affair can also help reduce any stress at home. Invite your loved ones to your BJJ training sessions, tournaments, and even classes so they can be a part of your journey. At a very minimum, share a few techniques with your family. Let them experience the power of BJJ and who knows, they might get hooked too. Jiu-Jitsu shouldn't feel like a mistress to your spouse. Imagine what it might look like. You leave, come home late, shower and pass out. Create some positive dialogue with your family about your training experiences.

Surround yourself with friends and family who value the importance of physical and mental exercise. You might even be able to recruit a friend to train with you. If not, befriend a teammate at your school. Ask them for their phone number and make them your "accountability partner."

An accountability partner is someone who will support and encourage you through your martial arts journey as you work toward your BJJ goals together. They can instill a sense of duty and elevate the experience, boosting your chances of actually achieving your goals. They can take the form of a family member who trains, a partner at your academy, or even an online friendship. The value is in the mutual support you can offer each other. Plus you may end up with a good friend too.

You can also create virtual friendships by joining online BJJ groups. We have a BJJ After 40 Private Facebook group. This is a great place to ask questions, share your experiences with others your age and more!

https://www.facebook.com/groups/354014296093221/?
ref=share_group_link

Just like the closed guard in BJJ, "time blocking" is another tried and true strategy that can help you successfully plan your day. With this method you allocate specific chunks of time throughout the day to work on individual projects.

The Pomodoro method is also very helpful for "getting a lot of shit done!" This aims to break tasks into small chunks called "Pomodoro's," followed by short breaks. The name comes from the Italian word for tomato. Think of a tomato shaped kitchen timer.

Here's how it works (by the way this is how I was able to complete three books in a year). Set a timer for 25-30 minutes. If you get interrupted during your work period, make a note, and continue the task. After the timer is completed, take a five minute break and begin a new Pomodoro. The goals is to complete four sessions with five minute breaks in between. You can use this method for studying BJJ notes, completing tasks outside

BJJ, watching and reviewing BJJ videos, etc.

Setting priorities is crucial for efficient time management. Just like you need a strategy to win a BJJ match, you also need to set priorities to keep your life in check. Like the four main positions in Jiu-Jitsu, create a hierarchy of key objectives. You'll be able to designate tasks more effectively and devote more time and energy where it is most needed.

Integrating BJJ into family life is rewarding and fun. Many gyms offer family sessions, consider enrolling together and learn as a unit. Simple home-based drills can turn into fun, bonding activities. Be sure to share what you learned in class and discuss the life lessons from BJJ.

The **Pareto Principle**, often known as the **80/20 rule**, states that a person's efforts typically only yield a positive return on investment of 20% of the time. This means that the majority of your success in BJJ will come from mastering a small set of fundamental techniques. Take this principle and apply it to your life by zeroing in on the activities that will have the greatest impact. You'll save time and energy, allowing you to devote more attention to things like family and BJJ.

Here's your top tips for balancing BJJ, work and family:

- You have to find your "no" voice. Realize your limitations and don't sign up for more than you can handle. Focus your efforts on the things that matter the most to you. If your partner doesn't train BJJ then find other workouts you can do together. (Hiking, walking, weight training, biking, etc.) This will take the stress off the time you are away from your family for BJJ.

- Using a calendar or planner can help you keep track of your training schedule. By putting your BJJ and weight training days into your calendar you're making a personal commitment to follow through. Plus it's a good idea to let your family know in advance when you're training. Mark BJJ into your daily, weekly and monthly calendar. Schedule your days in advance so that you may devote time to your workout, your job, and your family. Get into a regular regimen to ensure your consistency. Following a regular schedule that you adhere to is far better than being hot one week and cold the next.

- Goals for exercise, work, and family activities should be broken down into manageable daily, weekly, and monthly chunks. Remember, the way you eat an elephant is one bite at a time. Attack your goals in small, realistic, digestible chunks. If you went to BJJ class twice per week, every week for six months you would have decent results. But you might say, "That's not enough!" But then you had a buddy who trained 5-6 days per week. But about once per month he would miss 3-4 times because he was always "banged up." Who is better off in the long run? Slow and steady usually wins the race. Keep your training schedule easy and sustainable. You can always reevaluate as you go and add and subtract where it is needed.

- Finding yourself a training partner can be of great value. By having someone you can share a feedback loop with is essential. "A feedback loop is a process in which the output of a system is returned as input. In other words, it's a cycle of information that is continuously updated and used to modify a system's behavior." When you have a consistent training partner you can motivate each other. But you can also gain important data. You can collaborate with each other on 'what is' and isn't working. You will become a more well-rounded and adaptable BJJ practitioner by training with a partner who can help you adjust to diverse training settings and styles. The criticism you receive from your accountability partner will be honest and constructive, allowing you to see where you could make changes for the better. Plus it's important to have someone who knows your personal BJJ inside and out. I have rolled with my wife for many years (she's also a BJJ black belt). She's my toughest adversary on the mats because she knows my game better than I do!

Mission:

With this operation the goal is to align your personal, work and BJJ life cohesively together. Remember, the objective is to create a realistic, sustainable path that encompasses and benefits all aspects of your life. Too much of anything can be counterproductive. You want to strike the perfect balance between BJJ, work and family.

Create a weekly BJJ schedule that includes weight training. I believe that strength training for the over 40 practitioner is crucial. "A body without armor is inviting injury!" If your work schedule stays consistent from week to week, then build your training around it. If your schedule changes regularly, you'll have to make accommodations and adaptations. Remember, consistency is the key that unlocks potential. It's better to be slow and steady than hot and cold.

Along with your BJJ and weight training, you'll want to schedule in some Pomodoro's for BJJ study and review. This doesn't need to be anything to significant other than 15-20 minutes a few times per week. You can set a reminder in your phone for review sessions. What do you go over? Whatever you're working on in class. According to Pareto's principle, 80% of your BJJ submissions will come from 20% of your techniques. Build strength around what's working and address what is not. You can also use your study time to build other aspects of your game.

One of the best parts of BJJ is the friendships and sense of community. If you're new to your school, then it's time to make some friends! Don't run out the door after class, stay around and socialize. Often times you'll see small groups gathering and chatting after open mats or grappling. Build some courage and walk over and introduce yourself to the group. If you're a veteran of BJJ, take a moment and say hi to the new guy or gal starting class!

With this mission we encourage you to find an accountability partner. Simply exchange numbers with a teammate and text them outside of class. You can motivate one another, get together and drill or just have a new buddy who shares a similar interest.

Get your family involved! Try to share your joy of BJJ by coming home in the best mood ever. You can even show your kids and partner some of what you're learning. Just don't use them like a rag doll! But rather empower them with some BJJ that they can grasp. Who knows you might even get them to come to a class with you. At the very least, invite them to BJJ social events so they can experience the same joy you get from Jiu-Jitsu!

Men's Health

Jiu-Jitsu doesn't just keep us fit; it challenges us to be our best selves—mentally, emotionally, and physically. Reflect on the transformation you experience stepping off the mats: the shift from an awful mood to rejuvenation. It's this power of transformation that aligns with the martial artists vision of living with a deep sense of purpose. Training is our ultimate health insurance, an investment not just in bodily health but in our spiritual and emotional vigor.

As practitioners over 40, it's vital to maintain all systems and organs in optimal function. Regular screenings are part of this—think of them as maintaining and tuning your vehicle for a long journey. Your role in your family and community demands this attentiveness to health. Challenge yourself to upgrade not only your physical being but your inner self as well, integrating curiosity with mastery.

Have a deep appreciation for every interaction, understanding that each person you meet is here to enhance your practice. Think of each training partner as a teacher and a guide towards living your fullest life.

It's also essential to keep tabs on your fellow practitioners. Let them know their health matters to you, encouraging them to stay on the mats and engage with life fully. This is your way of extending your strength beyond the physical, offering support for mental health, this is crucial for a man's holistic development.

Managing health through different stages of life ensures a longer, happier practitioner. Adjust your diet to support your training intensity and physiological needs. Regular health screenings can catch potential issues early. Incorporate strength, flexibility, and cognitive exercises into your routine.

Mission :

Obtain a full body physical. Go beyond the basics: cholesterol, blood glucose levels, colon and prostate screenings, and cognitive checks. Adjust your diet to support your training intensity and life stage needs. Add strength, flexibility, and cognitive exercises to your routine to foster resilience against the natural aging process. Unapologetically take responsibility for being your own advocate for discussions on whole health topics with your primary care physician and take advantage of any possible secondary opinions. What resonates best with you?

Menstruation and Menopause

Let's be in this for the long haul and plan ahead, preferably the night before so whatever travels we take we're ready for the unexpected. That means an emergency kit is a must for any female to keep loaded up along with extra gear in her bag.

In my opinion, the specific physical exercise of BJJ is unlike anything else in the world for the mental and emotional wellbeing of a woman. It's really an easy way to track your training. How has the last month been and where do I intend to go in the near future? Just like you would modify your game if you had a nagging injury that you know was going to be coming back around you'll need to be creative at times and relentless in others to find ways to stay on the mats. I promise you'll get the return on your investment.

And let's not forget that iconic scene in the original "Anchorman," where Ron Burgundy, in his infinite wisdom, declares that women don't belong in the newsroom because it is "Anchorman, not Anchorlady!" Of course we don't have to share that same sentiment. Let guys show their support by being there to drill differently or tread a little lighter so you can train too.

Training through menstruation isn't just possible; it's empowering. Jiu-Jitsu gives you the strength to harmonize with your body's rhythms rather than battle against them. Slow down your skills, focus on step by step principle based learning and feeling good the whole way through sparring sessions and gently stretch.

As a woman transitions into menopause, the challenges evolve, but so does her strengths. Hot flashes and mood swings? Incorporate a cool-down period after training. Only allow light, moisture wicking materials on your body and dress in layers. Keep fans stashed everywhere, bring icepacks in your BJJ bag and always have a cold drink on hand.

Scientific studies suggest - okay, it was in "Anchorman" - that "their periods attract bears." While we laugh off such absurdities, it's crucial to acknowledge and adapt to the real changes our bodies undergo.

Training during these phases isn't just about staying active; it's about transforming our approach to Jiu-Jitsu to align with our body's needs.

Mission:

Adapt Training Intensity: Hormonal fluctuations can affect energy levels, so it's important to listen to your body and adjust the intensity of training accordingly. During menstruation, some women may need to scale back on intense sparring sessions due to discomfort or fatigue, while others might feel more capable. Menopause may bring hot flashes or sleep disturbances that also impact energy levels and recovery.

Focus on Flexibility and Mobility: As estrogen levels decline, especially during menopause, the risk of joint stiffness and injury can increase. Incorporate more flexibility and mobility exercises into your routine to improve range of motion and reduce the risk of injuries.

Hydration and Nutrition: Adequate hydration is crucial. Hormonal changes can affect hydration levels and how your body uses certain nutrients. Increase iron intake during menstruation if you experience heavy periods, and consider calcium and vitamin D supplements to support bone health during menopause.

Strength Training: Incorporate strength training to counteract the loss of muscle mass and bone density that can occur with hormonal changes in menopause. Weight-bearing exercises are particularly important to help maintain bone strength.

Psychological Support: Hormonal changes can also impact mood and mental health. Practices like yoga and meditation can be integrated into training to help manage stress, anxiety, and mood swings. A supportive training environment and community are invaluable.

Consult Health Professionals: Regular consultations with healthcare providers who understand the demands of BJJ can help manage symptoms and adjust health strategies effectively. This might include gynecologists, endocrinologists, or nutritionists.

Sexual Health

We've seen a lot over the years and yet it's one of the least talked about aspects of a practitioners' life. Your intimate relationships *will* effect your training. The 'for better or worse' part is entirely up to you.

Hormonal Balance: Sexual health influences hormonal levels, particularly testosterone in men and estrogen in women, which play crucial roles in muscle strength, bone density, and overall energy levels. Maintaining these hormones through healthy sexual practices helps ensure that you have the stamina and resilience needed for rigorous training sessions.

Mental Health and Mood: Regular sexual activity is linked to reduced stress and improved mood. The release of endorphins during sex acts as a natural stress reliever and mood enhancer, making it easier to handle the psychological pressures of training and competition.

Relationships and Emotional Support: Strong, healthy relationships contribute to emotional stability. For BJJ practitioners, having a supportive partner can provide emotional sustenance, which is particularly beneficial during challenging periods of training or when dealing with injuries. A healthy sexual relationship fosters intimacy and trust, creating a strong support network that extends beyond the mats.

Depression and Anxiety Management: Regular sexual activity is associated with lower rates of depression and anxiety. The physical and emotional closeness inherent in healthy sexual relationships helps in managing these conditions, which can otherwise negatively impact a practitioner's focus, motivation, and performance.

Social Connections and Longevity in Sport: Engaging in a community where relationships are nurtured, and mental health is prioritized can lead to longer, more satisfying careers in sports like BJJ. Practitioners who maintain strong interpersonal connections and manage their sexual and mental health effectively are more likely to enjoy their journey in the sport and persist through the ups and downs of training.

Mission:

Let your sexual vitality be a force that enhances not just your physical health, but your emotional and spiritual well-being, making every roll on the mats a reflection of your balanced, dynamic spirit.

Survival Expert: MARTY JOSEY

Marty started training in the martial arts over 30 year ago and over the years has studied various arts including Shorin Ryu Karate, Tae Kwon Do, Kenpo (Black Belt), Progressive Fighting Systems / Contemporary Jeet Kune Do (PFS) (Apprentice Instructor), Fear Adrenal Stress Response (FAST Defense-Certified instructor), Submission Grappling, and Gracie Jiu-Jitsu. He is currently a brown belt with four stripes in BJJ.

He is a certified Breath instructor, a certified Oxygen Advantage system instructor, and a certified Wim Hof method instructor.

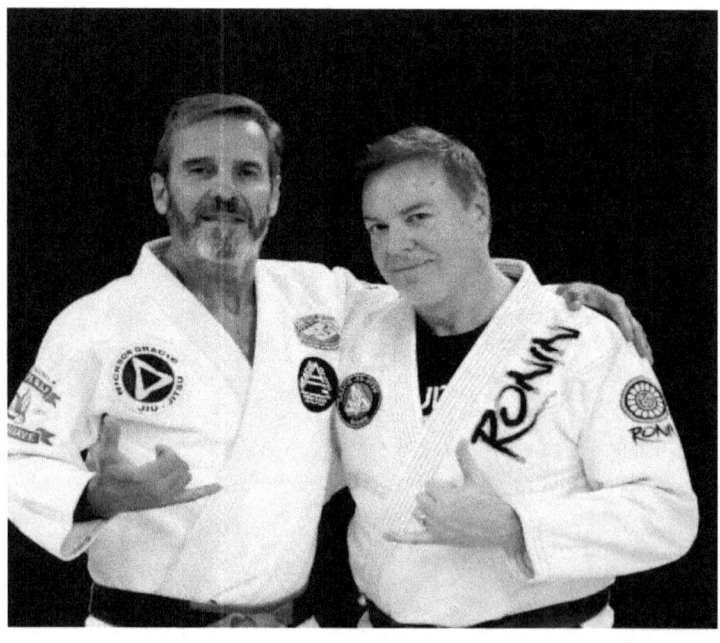

Intel:

In 2018 I had the privilege of meeting Marty in person when he came to visit me at my academy in Colorado. I did a video segment for over 40 practitioners for his BJJ and breathing program. We also did an interview for his "Gracie, Jiu-Jitsu Rocks" podcast.

Since we were close in age, we had a lot in common, and struck up a friendship that has continued to this day. Marty is a highly intelligent and compassionate person with a wealth of knowledge on BJJ and breath control. I am honored to have him share his experiences.

From the Source:

The biggest challenge facing older BJJ practitioners is that our lung capacity diminishes every year. Like all other physical attributes, such as muscular strength, speed, and recovery, our capacity to breathe is declining (and likely has already declined) so we are not at a level playing field with our younger counterparts.

Another challenge is that we all breathe (even if we are not aware of it, we still breathe), and because it's automatic, we tend to take it for granted. Because we take it for granted, we don't see a need to work on improving our breathing capacity. But just because we breathe naturally, it doesn't mean we are breathing anything close to optimally.

The two biggest problems I see in older BJJ practitioners (and practitioners in general) are:

1. Not regulating our breath (either over breathing or holding our breath)

2. Inability to stay calm (panicking under the pressure of bad positions). Over breathing (breathing too heavily or too fast) will sap our

energy very quickly. Holding our breath will do this as well. Not being able to stay calm under pressure will lead to a panicky feeling and evoke the stress response, leading to exhaustion as well. It is vital that we learn to regulate our breathing.

All of these are compounded when we get drawn into the action of matching our younger training partners' physical attributes and pace. So, not only is it vital to learn how to regulate our breathing, but we must learn to keep our egos out of it and do what's best for us, without focusing on winning.

Again, just because it's automatic does not mean we are breathing well. It doesn't mean we are breathing to our full functional capacity. To breathe optimally, we must breathe diaphragmatically. What exactly does this mean? We've all heard that we should use our diaphragm but how do we do this? What exactly is our diaphragm and how do we use it? Our diaphragm is a large muscle that sits in the middle of our torso. It actually separates our upper torso (our organs such as our heart, lungs, etc. and our lower torso (our organs such as our liver, stomach, intestines, etc.). It is attached to our sternum, our lower ribs, and our spine. When at rest it sits coiled up and when contracted (when we breathe correctly, it flattens out and lowers several inches. This creates a negative air pressure and causes air to be pulled down into the lower lobes of our lungs, where more of the "magic" (gas exchange) happens.

The best way to understand this is in terms of breathing vertically or horizontally. If we breathe vertically, we rise or get taller as we inhale, we are using our upper chest, shoulder, and neck muscles to breathe. These should be accessory muscles, helping out when we need them during times of severe exertion. If we use them as primary breathing muscles, we can develop issues in our neck and shoulders, as well as gas out much more quickly. This is easy to fall into a dysfunctional habit because our lungs are in our chest cavity, it's natural to think we're supposed to breathe in our upper chest. Now think back to having a check up at the Dr's office and they place a stethoscope on your chest and upper back and ask you to breathe. In reality, breathing vertically is a very inefficient way to breathe and by contrast breathing horizontally (your torso actually widens instead of lengthens) when you inhale, is a much more efficient method of breathing.

The initial way to learn and develop lower torso (diaphragmatic) breathing is through belly breathing. When you inhale, you move your belly out and when you exhale your belly moves inward. Eventually with practice, you can develop the ability to breathe all the way around your torso. Then when you inhale, your torso (ribs) moves out in all directions like a small umbrella opening out from the center of your torso. This not only means more functional breathing in general, but leads you to many more options on the mat. This is when things get interesting.

Breath work training will increase your ability to regulate your breathing. It will give you the ability to produce more energy when needed and produce calmness when needed. Let me give you an example of when and how this is important. Although I'm not an avid competitor, about four years ago I decided to compete at the BJJ Masters Worlds. I used specific breath work extensively in my training. On the day of the competition, when my nerves were firing and my anxiety level was increasing, I used focused breathing to calm my nerves while waiting for my matches. Then, during warm up and right before my matches I used another type of breathing to increase my energy. This got me ready physically and psychologically. During my matches I focused on regulating my breath, and after / between matches I down regulated my breathing to recover faster. I really believe that breathing was my "secret weapon" that helped me be successful taking home the gold. Of course, one's technique is extremely important, but I really believe that if power and skill are comparable, the conditioning (breathing) can be the decisive factor.

One breathing strategy that's very useful in rolling or competition is what I call the **Soda Can principle (or analogy)**. If you pick up a can of soda and try to squeeze / smash it, it's pretty impossible. But if you open it up and pour out the soda, then try to squeeze it, you'll find that you can crush it very easily. That's because the stabilizing pressure is no longer there. The liquid was giving the can stability.

Our breathing is like this as well. If, for example, we are on the bottom of a large opponent (say in cross side position) and we make the mistake of letting too much of our air out, the weight of the person will smash us and "take up the space." Then when we try to take another breath we will find that we are unable to inhale and thus will feel smothered and crushed.

Therefore, we need to keep a certain amount of air in our thoracic cavity, while we focus on breathing. This should consist of short, smooth exhales. By focusing on the exhales we will ensure that we are not holding our breath, and by keeping a certain amount of air in our lungs we'll ensure that we can't be smashed and sapped of our ability to breathe.

Also, remember me talking about breathing all the way around the torso? When you develop this skill, you can easily breathe in all positions you find yourself in. For example you're on the bottom of cross side position, and your opponent is lying heavily across your chest. You can't breathe into the front of your torso but it's okay. You simply breathe into a pocket on the side of your torso (by expanding your ribs outward). You're able to maintain your breathing and stay calm until you can execute your next move.

Another tip: Become aware of your opponent's / training partner's breathing. It gives you valuable information. If you hear them over breathing or breathing hard, it lets you know they are wearing down, and it may be your time to turn up the intensity, etc.

How can proper breathing improve breathing and stamina for older BJJ athletes?

Proper breathing builds lung capacity, strengthens and tones breathing muscles, such as your diaphragm, your obliques, your rectus abdominis, and your intercostal muscles (muscles between and attaching to your ribs).

Everyone thinks that just doing more cardio will do the trick and be enough for them, but it's not. It can certainly help, and cardio is amazing for increasing circulation and for building cardiac performance but if your blood doesn't have optimal O2 in it, the circulation that you have won't deliver the amount of O2 to the cells that it could have. Oxygen is cell fuel and we need it more than anything. It's what gives us energy.

Cardio also doesn't optimize your lung function or improve the flexibility of your thoracic cavity (bones, cartilage, tendons, and muscles that make up your chest wall). It doesn't strengthen your breathing muscles (inhale and exhale muscles) or your diaphragm. In fact, in the words of Dr. Belisa Vranich, "you could have the heart and cardiovascular system of an elite athlete but the lungs and breathing muscles of a couch potato."

Unless we've specifically trained our breathing muscles, they tend to exhaust way before our other muscles do (quads, arms, etc.). Because of this we don't get a good enough work out for them by just doing cardio.

Regular breathing training increases your breathing skill and capacity, and serves as "insurance" for when we need it. It's like a breathing bank account. The more we deposit (regular breathing training), the more capacity we have. When we need to make a withdrawal (expending a lot of energy, say in a tough training session or a competition) the more we have to use.

Can you explain the connection between breathing and stress management in high pressure BJJ situations, particularly for older athletes?

Without getting too in depth here, the somatic part of our nervous system is divided into two parts: the sympathetic and the parasympathetic nervous branches. The sympathetic is responsible for fight or flight and the parasympathetic is responsible for "rest and digest." Competitions tend to be stressful situations for most of us. Our fight or flight mechanism is usually evoked and we're ready for action. But we are also on overdrive and this can lead us to quick burn out. During these times we need to be able to down regulate and calm down. We need to be able to find the right level of fight or flight to be useful and the right amount of "chill" to be able to handle the situation clearly and calmly. The great thing about breath work training is that you become more capable of tapping into which part of your nervous system you want to be tap into and which mental state you want to be in.

A strategy that can be extremely helpful with developing our ability to remain calm under pressure is to put ourselves into difficult and uncomfortable situations. By doing this consistently, we develop a certain comfort level by just being there often. Focus on surviving the position and developing the feeling that you're going to be okay there. Usually by the time someone has progressed into high ranks, this has been developed at least to some extent, and practitioners that are less experienced find these "smothering" positions extremely terrifying (when you can't breath, it's natural to panic). However, even for the more experienced practitioners who have developed some capacity to stay calm, I have found that if they work specifically on their breathing related to these positions, they get to a much higher level of comfort. The best way to train yourself to endure these positions is to spend time there but most importantly to focus on your breathing while there. Going back to the soda can analogy, practicing holding some breath in your torso (chest and ribs), while exhaling out and enduring these positions develops your comfort and capacity to become more comfortable in these positions. And when you're not having to panic, you can focus on your logical steps to improve your position (without opening yourself up to an attack or submission).

By training yourself to stay calm and to tap into the parasympathetic nervous system, you are able to regulate your breathing and conquer the situation.

How can older BJJ athletes incorporate breathing techniques into their daily routine, both on and off the mat?

Okay for "off" the mat, generally the focus needs to be on stimulating the parasympathetic nervous system. This is because most of us are generally more stressed and keyed up on a daily basis than is healthy. There are so many stressors in modern day life, so we need to focus on lowering stress. This is accomplished in simple terms by slowing our breathing down and making our exhales longer than our inhales. You can experiment with different ratios but make sure the exhales are longer.

For performance (on the mat), breathing capacity needs to be increased. My advice to accomplish this is to adopt a specific breathing workout program.

This should be a separate breathing program from any other work out. The aim of this program would be to build and strengthen your breathing muscles and your functional capacity to breathe. Imagine taking your breathing muscles out of your body and working them out separately. Then, after you have developed their function and capacity, putting them back into your body. It's like getting a lung transplant. Not really, but you get my drift here. It's like supercharging your system.

The next part (for either on or off the mat progress) is to focus on your ongoing maintenance for the long term. This part could be included in your current morning routines (mobility, mediation, etc). Whatever you're currently do as a morning routine (and if you don't currently have a morning routine I highly suggest you start one. It sets the stage for your day and literally programs you for a positive, happy, and successful day. You can add some specific breathing / breath work training into it too.

After you've built your breathing capacity, it's easy to maintain it. It doesn't take much time to keep things at a great level, and remember as we age our capacity naturally declines so it is vital that we build and maintain our functional breathing capacity.

It's literally the most effective thing I've ever done for my Jiu-Jitsu as well as my life and health in general. Once you breathe better and more optimally, it affects every area of your life. You feel better, perform better, and are in control of boosting your energy at will or relaxing your mind and body exactly when you need it. It's the most powerful thing I've ever learned and done for myself and it's brought back a high level of joy to my Jiu-Jitsu. It has helped me "play" and operate at a much higher level (psychologically, emotionally, and spiritually) in my everyday life.

Sleep

Let's start with the most important form of recovery, sleep! You can't sleep? As a dad of four kids, with a set of toddler twins, I know the feeling. You've probably been there too. (Maybe in a different way) Your muscle and joints ache from a tough night on the mats. Your brain is spinning from learning new moves, tapping people and getting tapped. You want to sleep even more than you desire food. Your bed is calling your name. But you simply can't sleep. We all experience the phenomena where sleep becomes more essential and elusive as we age. But in order to recover properly, keep your wits about you and maintain your competitive edge, you need to sleep.

One of the greatest recovery tools is one they we know and love, sleep. Remember the days when you could go to the gym, pull an all nighter with your buddies, and still show up for work the next day? Well those days are long gone my friend. As we age, our bodies require more time to repair itself. We then add Jiu-Jitsu to the mix and we face a unique set of circumstances. Sleep is our bodies system for repairing itself. Plus if you miss sleep often enough you risk becoming the "grumpy old person." (And nobody has time for that)

In addition to repairing our BJJ-worn bodies, sleep also helps with memory and cognitive function. Grappling is an intensely memory-based martial art. Where striking arts are based on a smaller set of movements. Grappling arts work from two sets of limbs on two partners. The possibilities become more complicated and overwhelming.

If you want to keep your BJJ brain sharp, sleep is essential. "You snooze, you lose." In this case if you don't snooze, you really lose! Rest is truly a magical elixir. It helps with testosterone production, mood and hormonal regulation, clears brain fog, relieves muscle soreness and inflammation.

When you sleep your body also produces collagen. Experts say that during the third and fourth stages of sleep our body goes into repair mode. This is where the important work is done. But if we cannot get a restful nights sleep, then we create a host of problems for ourselves. BJJ training is hard enough, why make it more challenging. Remember, a well-rested grappler is a dangerous grappler!

But how do you set the conditions for a good nights sleep? Well like most things you will have a better experience if you create the right "set and set-ting." Whenever possible have a regular bedtime and waking time to bet-ter sync your circadian rhythms. You have to resist the urge for late night BJJ viewing on YouTube. The blue light emitted from your screen time can disrupt your natural sleep. If you're like me and you need to fall asleep to a 90's TV classic like "Cheer's." Then turn the screen down and listen to your favorite classic television show. Better yet, turn off the electronics and curl up with a nice book. Perhaps that's what you're doing right now with this informative read.

Black out curtains are a great way to decrease light and prepare your body for rest. I also like to use a sound machine as well. White noise has shown to help with sleep. It is a type of sound that contains all of the audible frequencies. It can help to mask other sounds like traffic or unruly dogs. Some people describe the consistent sound of white noise to being like a lullaby. Studies have shown that white noise can also help synchronize brain waves. This can be helpful in the organization of new information and consolidation of memories.

But before your body even hits the mattress make sure your body is ready for sleep. A warm bath after a tough evening of training can be the perfect path to a restful nights sleep. Epson salts in the bath can be a great way to alleviate any inflammation. Epsom salt, (magnesium sulfate) has been used for centuries as a remedy and to alleviate soreness. Some believe that the bath is an excellent way for your body to absorb the magnesium. You can also use the time to mentally rep out what you've learned in class. This will help get any mental BJJ baggage out of your head before it hits the pillow. Just like it helps to exhaust your physical body, you also want to tire your active BJJ mind.

Avoid any stimulating activities like tv's, computers or doing work before bed. Limiting caffeine and alcohol consumption in the evenings can be beneficial to good sleep. You'll also want to steer clear of eating a full meal before bed. Consuming a lot of food can cause discomfort and indigestion when you sleep. You may also find that when you eat before bed the increased metabolic activity from digestion can make it difficult to fall asleep.

Meditation can also provide a great path to a good nights sleep. Research has shown that it can enhance melatonin production which can significantly improve the quality of sleep. It can also increase alpha brain waves, which are associated with a state of calmness and relaxation.

Make sure you have a comfortable clean bed. By taking the time to make your bed each day you prepare yourself for sleep each night. A clean, made bed is far more inviting than a pile of tangled blankets and sheets.

A temperature of between 60 and 67 degrees Fahrenheit are recommended by sleep experts. They say that people sleep best in this temperature range because it facilitates thermoregulation, which in turns creates more restful sleep (Thermoregulation is the process by which your body maintains a comfortable temperature while sleeping) The core body temperature drops in the first few hours of sleep and slowly rises as dawn approaches. A warm room will cause you to awaken. **Keep it cool and you'll sleep like a baby!**

Mission:

Go to bed and wake up at the same time whenever possible. (Even weekends) Make your bedroom conducive to sleep by keeping it cool, dark, quiet and comfortable. Invest in a mattress and pillow that you love! Steer away from caffeine and alcohol before bed. Naps, if taken, should be limited to no more than thirty minutes. Always nap during sunlight, never in the evening. Regular exercise helps promote sleep. Stretch and move your body before bed. Avoid computers, phones and the television while you're in bed. The blue light disrupts sleep.

Meditation - Listen to one of our guided meditations before bed. Keep a notepad next to your bed if you are awakened. You can track when you wake up by keeping notes. You can also use it to capture ideas or thoughts when you awaken.

Foods that help you sleep: Tart cherries - a source of melatonin, Kiwi - a source of serotonin - which can regulate sleep patterns, Almonds - high in magnesium - which helps with relaxation and muscle soreness, Warm milk - Contains tryptophan, and amino acids that induces sleep, Bananas - a good source of magnesium and potassium, Herbal teas - Lavender teas, chamomile and valerian root all promote better sleep.

Stretches that help promote relaxation and sleep:

Butterfly stretch - Sit on the floor with your bottoms of your feet pressed together, and your heels pulled towards your groin area. Gently press your knees towards the floor and hold for 30-60 seconds.

Seated forward bend - Sit on the floor with your legs extended forward and pressed together. Point your toes skyward as you bend forward and reach for your toes.

Child's pose - Begin on your hands and knees and then lower your hips down towards your heels, gently stretching your arms forward. You can rest your forehead on the floor. You can also reach your arms behind your back as you bend forward.

Debriefing Assessment:

Reflect on how you manage the interplay between your BJJ training, family commitments, and professional responsibilities. Evaluate the strategies you use to ensure each area receives adequate attention without compromising the others. How do you prioritize your time, and what challenges have you faced in maintaining this balance? Consider the support systems you have in place and any adjustments that might improve your overall life balance.

Assess your approach to nutrition and weight management in the context of your BJJ training and lifestyle needs. How do you align your dietary habits with your training goals and weight categories for competition? Reflect on the effectiveness of your current nutrition strategies and consider any changes that could enhance your performance and health.

This section invites you to consider broader health topics that are pertinent to training but often overlooked. Reflect on how issues related to men's health, menstruation, and menopause affect your training or the training of others in your BJJ community. Assess the awareness and sensitivity within your gym regarding these issues and explore ways to support inclusivity and understanding.

Evaluate how you maintain sexual health and its relationship to your overall physical and mental well-being. Consider the role of physical fitness, including BJJ training, in promoting a healthy sexual life. Reflect on any educational resources or discussions within your training community about maintaining sexual health.

Sleep is crucial for recovery and performance in BJJ. Reflect on your sleep habits and their impact on your training effectiveness and daily functioning. Assess whether you are getting adequate rest and if not, identify potential reasons and solutions to improve your sleep quality.

Operations:

Non Existent

Explore innovative recovery methods beyond
conventional techniques, including cutting-edge
therapies and psychological resilience strategies.
This section is vital for overcoming plateaus and
rejuvenating your training approach.

Scan the QR code for techniques on managing unseen challenges.

https://www.youtube.com/playlist?list=PLwb5iQup993_
MmzfOHOTUGhUyfNXETeBR

Injury Prevention

L et's define "Sustainability" as it relates to BJJ practice after 40 years old. *"How can I fulfill my current needs without compromising my future needs?"*

It's not so much a definition as it is an important question. But the answer to this question will pave your future in BJJ. The point of beginning your training was not to get hurt, have multiple surgeries and be chronically sore. Nor was the point so you could tap out a 20 year old purple belt. (Although that does sound like fun) Maybe you wanted to get in better shape, learn something new, meet people, become a ninja. Regardless of your reason, you didn't do it to mangle up your body.

So how do we create a sustainable path that doesn't throw all the fun out the window? As we age our natural recovery process begins to slow down. It becomes more important than ever to address recovery in an active real way. It can't just be you get a massage every so often because you're sore. Or worse, the chronic soreness leads to an injury. The healing part of your training is just as important as the time on the mats.

This means you have a plan and a path to feeling better. Just like you schedule your training, you need to plan out your recuperation time. Without relief, "bumps and bruises" begin to pile up and lead to chronic injuries. The tennis elbow left unattended becomes a future injury. Aching bodies and injuries mean more time off from the mats. Plus nobody wants to be in pain!

For a forty plus grappler I generally recommend no more than 3-4 BJJ training days per week. Yes we all want to roll more, including me. But I too have to exercise my discipline and try to only roll on my rolling days. Of course I would love it every day, but it's not sustainable for my age. My path, like yours, has to outlive the present moment.

A great schedule could be three days of BJJ training, with 2-4 days of weight training. Building strength is one of the best ways to prevent an injury. Having a strong, resilient body will get you through those tough rolls mostly unscathed.

Possible Training Schedule:

Monday - BJJ

Tuesday - Weight Training

Wednesday - R & R

Thursday - BJJ

Friday - Weight Training

Saturday - BJJ

Sunday - R & R or Light weights

*You can arrange and rearrange the days in a way that fits into your schedule. Do your best to spread it out. I always try to schedule an "R & R" day between tough training days. Don't try to "push through the pain." Listen to your body first and foremost. You're the expert of your own body. On your rest and recovery days you should be moving your body. This could be a light stretch, walk / hike / bike, yoga, etc. In addition, choose one recovery option for each R & R day.

Options for recovery: (choose one for each Rest & Recovery day)

Massage - Deep tissue massage is perfect for BJJ. The therapist will be able to relieve deep knots and any tension you may be carrying.

Acupuncture - I have personally have had great success using it for chronic tennis elbow.

Foam Rolling - Is a form of self - myofascial release. The roller will help you break up any deep rooted tightness.

Massage Gun - This is another form of myofascial release. The massage gun can be used on trigger points for pain relief.

Cupping - Has roots in Chinese medicine. Glass cups are placed on your body and the suction causes skin and muscle to pulled into it. This causes increased blood flow and pain relief. Cupping can also improve circulation and decrease inflammation.

Cold plunge / Ice bath - If you can handle the cold, many people speak of great results with ice baths. Just look on social media and you'll see video after video of people freezing their asses off in ice water. Just remember, you don't have to post a video or picture for it to work.

Cryotherapy - I've never used this method for recovery. However, users claim to have decreased muscle soreness, reduced inflammation and improved circulation.

Epsom Salt Bath (heat) - This involves soaking in warm water filled with epsom salts (magnesium sulfate). Proponents believe that it decreases inflammation from the absorption of magnesium into your body. (There's no hard evidence to prove or disprove it) But it does seem to help with relaxation and soreness. I have found that epsom baths do relieve soreness and are great for self-reflection or for repping out a few extra BJJ moves!

Mindful Meditation - This form of meditation involves focusing your attention on the present moment. It includes observing: What your thoughts are doing, how your body feels, physical sensations, emotional state, etc. This can help to reduce stress, improve body awareness and create a sense of calmness. You can also use it to visualize BJJ sequences and steps of moves to further anchor them into your mind.

Stretching outside - By taking your stretching outside (weather permitting - although it can be fun to stretch in the snow) you have an opportunity to connect with nature. By being outside you create a "grounding" effect that connects you to the earth. You may find that being outside breathing the fresh air feels amazing and can have calming effect. Plus the sunlight can give you a vitamin D boost! It is important to note that you should look at the air quality in your area to make sure you aren't negating the benefits of exercise.

EGO

Jiu-Jitsu for me is about efficiency of movement. When you tend to rely on strength or speed alone, what do you do when the gas tank is on empty? The answer is, you move worse than before and you begin to make poor choices. This now creates further risk for both partners.

How do we improve technique? First you have to admit that you have a problem. Say it aloud, "I, state your name, cannot exercise my internal self-discipline and am addicted to using strength and speed. I realize that this is a problem and I am ready to address it." Great job! Now we can begin our work here.

I'm only somewhat kidding here. Sometimes we don't realize that we are going "H.A.M." on someone. Or in some cases, we keep getting hurt but we can't understand why? Maybe we go so hard that we invite our partners to one up us. Instead of a good, fluid roll we create a "tug of war." This can be especially dangerous for two, newer inexperienced over 40 white belts.

"Leave your ego at the door" You've probably seen or heard this saying as it relates to BJJ. The idea being that you don't need your ego to practice Jiu-Jitsu. The implication is that if you were to engage in such activities on the mats, either you or a partner could be injured. The ego is fundamentally about self-identity, encompassing the sense of 'I' and 'me' as distinct from others. It's this self-governing sense of autonomy that drives our instinct for survival. This is crucial to our caveman brain. This is also important for social interactions. The ego also serves to aid us in decision making by allowing us to make good choices based upon emotional, practical, and moral considerations.

In the context of BJJ a weak or fragile ego would break under the constraints of being repeatedly tapped or "losing." A stronger ego allows for resilience and a competitive edge. The desire to improve, adapt and overcome is often the result of the ego. When is it too much? When you put "winning" and "tapping someone" ahead of their mental and physical safety.

Black belts in BJJ often talk about reaching a state of flow where their actions and reactions become automated, fluid, and instinctual. What they're really talking about is reaching a state of "egoless-ness," where the focus is purely on the present moment, free from the ego's influence.

I have always believed that white belts SHOULD leave their ego's at the door. Blue and purple belts however need them to advance forward. At this point the student understands the art far more deeply and can be trusted with their ego. But understand that this isn't the same ego as when they were a white belt, or no belt. They now see BJJ through a more mature lens. At purple belt you're beginning to master your BJJ sense of self identity. What will you be good at? What are your strengths, etc.? Purple belt are like teenage lions. No longer cubs, they need to be a little competitive with each other. They'll nip, bite and wrestle like their animal counterparts. This will serve them individually and elevate the collective group.

At brown belt we begin to diminish the ego as it is no longer an important part of the equation. The final colored belt in BJJ is about maturity and collaboration. Brown belts often begin to teach more and are expected to share the art with others. A good teacher will free themselves from the constraints of the ego to serve the higher good of themselves and their students. An ego-driven teacher is easy to spot. They tend to hoard their knowledge and roll hard on their students. (Or not at all) They will often use promotions and belts to control others. The world of BJJ is filled with many wonderful people, but with every bushel you're bound to find one or two rotten apples.

If you're not sure if you go too hard, ask your training partners. Another good clue is, are you constantly getting banged up. This can mean bruises, cuts, black eyes, lacerations, etc. Elbows and knees happen when we are being unmindful during a roll. Slow things down and you'll see more opportunities and less injuries.

Your breathing is often the first red flag that you're going to hard or too fast. By establishing an agreed upon slower pace with your partner before the roll can be helpful. Don't be vague either, give them a number to work with. "Let's go 20, 30, 40% when we roll." The challenge is for both of you to respect the boundaries you've set. With some partners you just won't be able to set perimeters. Maybe you're at an open mat and are unfamiliar with your partners. In those cases you have to closely monitor your own breathing.

One great tip is to breathe from the diaphragm, not from the chest. Think of when you are startled or scared. In those instances, we breathe from the chest which can causes shallow breathing. This means you're getting less oxygen with each inhalation. This can increase the feeling that you're drowning in your breath. This can cause a sense or fear, anxiety and panic for some people. When you breathe exclusively through your mouth and upper chest it triggers the parasympathetic nervous system which is responsible for "fight or flight."

With new white belts this is generally the biggest "cardio challenge" they face. The "real obstacle" they encounter isn't conditioning as much as it is understanding there's no reason to associate fear with a grappling match. Sitting here right now in a conscious, logical setting you might agree. But when you roll that mindset can fly right out the window.

Yes, there is value in being smashed and having to suffer through it. It builds grit and mental toughness. The eventual path out of suffering is through efficient breathing. Everything works and feels better when you can get air. BJJ is a game of physical chess. It's filled with riddles, puzzles and complexities that change constantly. This is part of the draw and fun of grappling. But how can you possibly solve these complex physical equations without support from your breath. The answer is that you cannot. Imagine sprinting one hundred yards and being handed a complicated math equation to solve as you're trying to catch your breath? You would probably get agitated and angrily say, get out of my face!

Here are some tips for improving your BJJ breathing:

- **Find your rhythm** - Don't get out of breath or worse try to "catch your breathe." Good breathing should feel natural and not forced. But you need to guide it in the right direction. Sometimes pacing your breath with your partners can be useful. Especially if you're a beginner and they're more advanced. Listen to their breathing and try to match it (unless they're suffering too, then just try and survive).

- **Stay loose and relaxed** - Don't tense or tighten your body. This forces you to burn energy and breathe harder. Plus a tense tight body is more apt to be injured.

[283]

- **Check-in with yourself** - Beginners often get trapped in a cyclone of chaos. Literally spinning out of control. This happens because we "lose ourselves" and go into a "lizard brain," "fight or flight" response. A mental check-point can slow everything down. If you get stuck in a position, here's your new mantra: Literally say this to yourself: "If I can breathe, I am alive. If I'm alive, I can think. If I can think, I can problem solve my way out of anything." The point is that you start with a mental check-in which leads to conscious breathing, which allows for a more informed experienced. You can think of consciousness as awareness. When someone says, "He has a high level of consciousness." Think of that as simply awareness, or access to better information. When you're more informed, you can make better decisions. Now apply this to your grappling. Better awareness leads to better breathing. This in turn allows for more conscious decision making. You're not just reacting, but controlling and dancing with the outcome. Not becoming a victim to it.

- **Improve your cardiovascular conditioning** - You don't need to be an olympic level athlete. But you do have to have a decent baseline cardio. If you're out of shape, then you need to start from there. This doesn't necessarily mean more rounds either. Instead of more rolling, you can add longer rounds. Conversely, you can also do shorter rounds with an emphasis on moving faster for short sprints, with short rests in between. Think of each dominant position as a rest stop. Maybe you use a short burst to pass the guard, establish control, then rest and recoup. Remember, you can't sprint a marathon. You also cannot jog or walk a marathon either. The objective is too strike a balance between rest and advancement of position with a controlled, favorable outcome. You can't move the entire time, nor can you rest the whole time either.

- **Practice breathing** - It always sounds funny to practice something that seems to run on auto-pilot our whole life. Now here we are training BJJ and it doesn't seem to be working right?! Like anything that you want to improve upon, you have to practice it. Pressure training can work well. This is where you purposely put yourself in positions where you have to escape while maintaining control of your cardio. You can also begin to address mindful breathing through a meditation practice.

Belly breathing -

Your diaphragm is a large dome-shaped muscle that expands when your breathe. It allows you to take large, full breaths. How does one belly breathe? Start in a comfortable position, place your hand on your stomach. Take slow, deep inhalations through your nose and slowly release the air through your mouth. Feel the rise and fall of your abdomen as you breathe. You can also practice by breathing in through the nose and then exhaling through the nose. You can also explore "nostril breathing." With this method, you breathe in through one nostril, hold it briefly and then release it through the other nostril. The process can then be reversed. This can have both a calming and balancing effect on the body.

Schedule breathing -

Set a daily alarm in your phone calendar to practice breath work for five minutes each day. Having a daily routine will create a habit.

Try different methods each time -

Nostril breathing, belly breathing, 4-7-8 breathing technique) With the 4-7-8 method you do the following: Breathe in through your nose for a count of 4, hold the breath for 7 seconds, exhale through your mouth for an 8 second count. Maintain the 4-7-8 count through the entire phase (inhale, hold, exhale). This can help to reduce stress, anxiety and have a calming effect.

Having an efficient breath when you roll not only saves you from cardio hell, it will also keeps you off the injured list! Poor breathing creates impaired focus. You simply can't make good decisions when you can't breathe. So with fatigue comes poor judgement. Exhaustion can compromise your ability to use good technique which can further lead to injury. There's nothing that demands your attention like getting control of your breath.

*We further expand on breathing with Survival Expert, Marty Josey!

Mission:

Let's start with one important new rule: warm ups are nonnegotiable. If your school doesn't do a strong warm up, you may have to do a little bit at home. Your body needs time to adapt to the conditions of BJJ. Not warming up and then training hard will surely lead to an injury. Create a set of movements that support both your BJJ and current physical condition. If for example you tend to have a tight back or shoulders. You need to make sure you properly warm those areas before arriving for class.

It's okay to say 'no' to someone who asks you to roll. If you don't feel safe and are at risk for injury, then "no thanks" is really the only option. I'm not recommending that you avoid the challenges of BJJ. Embrace the tough stuff, but avoid the "Crazy, spazzy partners." Remember, going home better than when you left is always the number one goal.

Be sure that you are not the crazy one either! The ego sometimes has a way of protecting our feelings. The brain has a powerful defense mechanism that uses repression, denial, or rationalization to guard us from uncomfortable feelings. Sometimes we think everyone else is going too hard, but in fact we could be equally or totally contributing to it ourselves. If you're a white belt, leave your ego at the door. Blue and purple belts can begin to employ it in a healthy supportive manner. For brown and black belts it's time to move on from the ego and make a shared impact within your BJJ community.

For beginners, the way we leave our ego at the door is recognizing the larger picture. We can't do BJJ alone, therefore it's important to not kill and destroy yourself and your training partners. If you break your toys, nobody gets to play! White belts should tap early on everything, especially the stuff you're not familiar with.

A good mantra is, "when you're trapped, tap!" This will keep you safe in unfamiliar territory. Try to find a good rhythm with your breath and never let it get away from you. When you can't breathe you are at greater risk for injury. Stay calm, relaxed and focus on employing good technique when you're grappling.

Also begin to build a good baseline of cardio so you're not winded when you're training. You don't want to rely solely on endurance anymore than you want to rely mainly on strength. Try to focus on good technique with a sprinkle of endurance and muscle.

Create mental check-points when you're rolling. These will allow you to mentally ground yourself in the present moment and get you out of your "fight or flight, lizard brain." Remember, a conscious brain is an aware brain. One that can strategize, out-wit and out perform others under hostile conditions. The phrase "an out of breath body leads to an out of sorts brain" highlights the importance of managing your physical exertion. Overexertion can lead to fatigue, which in turn affects mental clarity and decision-making skills. It's important to pace yourself, conserve energy when necessary, and recognize when to apply strength and when to relax.

Ultimately relaxation comes from efficient breathing. Begin a daily five minute breathing practice. (Set a reminder in your phone right now) Explore some of the different breathing methods mentioned like: 4-7-8, nostril, belly breaths, mindfulness meditation and more. At the minimum at least bring awareness to your breath. This will allow you to refocus your breathing pattern before it becomes erratic and uncontrolled.

Don't forget your breathing mantra: "If I can breathe, I am alive. If I'm alive, I can think. If I can think, I can problem solve my way out of anything." You don't need much space to breathe. When you're stuck in side control, think of yourself as a ninja underwater, breathing through a bamboo straw. If you stay calm, you will be fine; panic, and you will die. Just one inch of space can quickly become two with a slight shift of the body. This is how you calmly maneuver your way out of precarious situations, one inch at a time.

Recovery

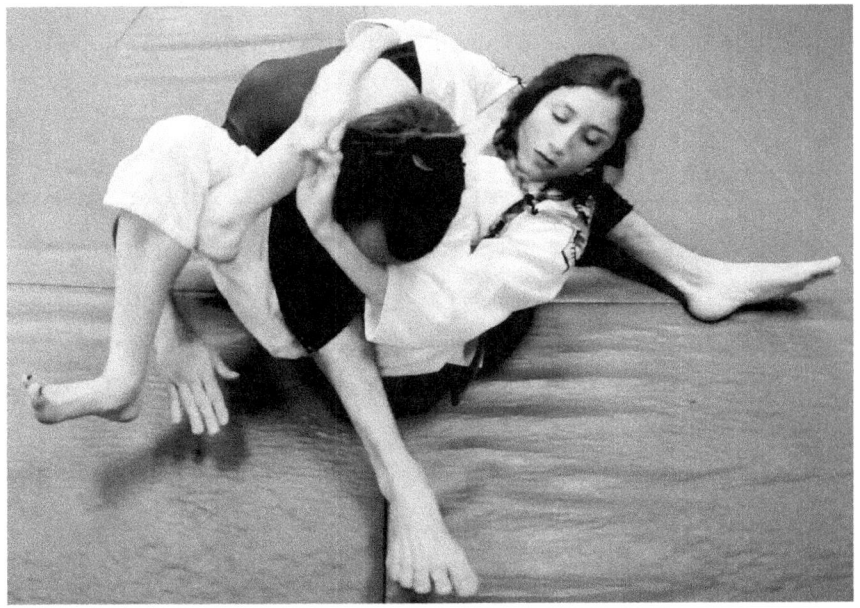

Sheena Bidwell, First Degree BJJ Black Belt

Recovery isn't just about getting back to where you were; it's about transforming into something even better.

Identify Your Current Strengths:

Post-injury or during a life upheaval, assess what you can do, not what you can't. Maybe you can't train physically, but you can improve your tactical knowledge or help coach newer students.

Adapt Techniques to Your Situation:

If certain moves are off-limits, find others that can be adapted to your current condition. Focus on upper body grips or lower body movements that don't strain your injured parts.

Mimic Successful Strategies:

Look at athletes who have faced similar challenges. How did they adapt? What new strategies did they employ? Mimic these approaches and make them your own.

Stay Connected:

Even if you can't train, stay involved. Mental and emotional engagement is a crucial part of recovery. My style of approach may be vastly different from yours, and for good reason. Just like when we grapple, to each their own. Before you read further, remove any and all distractions. Give this your full attention. Take 30 seconds up to two minutes before you read to breathe deep and sit with the awareness that you are consciously choosing to partake in your wellbeing.

Let's get physical: Meta-physical that is. We'll start by stripping down past the flesh, muscles and bones to the chakras and meridian centers. I'd recommend taking control of your energy, your vibe and essence. The way in which your mind listens to your heart then demands your body take action. Meaning, if all we can control in life is our attitude, might I suggest that of a warrior? One maybe marked with battle scars on the outside but a heart of gold on the inside for no other reason than the choice, that thought turned action, to keep going.

There may come a time where all you can move is your mind. Or direct your thoughts in a different direction.

Continually guide yourself to think thoughts of only everything working out for you and add the corresponding adjectives to imagine yourself living this life. This may sound something like "My back is flexible, I have a strong core, my training is going good, everything is working out for me." Keep it casual and content. Although your physical body may be keeping you in pain, your mind can free you.

Start with your breath. Breathing before any body movement. Deep and with your diaphragm moving as much of your belly as possible. This is where and when you can start practicing control. With mastery of your inner space it has no choice but to spill out. Be intentional. Practice alternate nostril breathing. Eventually you'll take your training to the mats and be able to keep a steady, relaxed breathing pattern in any position, during any transition and under any condition.

You have to decide and double down daily. Commit. Promise. Bind your identity to this choice. Ask yourself "Am I ready to heal?" Most likely, the answer is no. Your mind will yell yes! As your heart quietly whispers the truth, it needs tender loving care. It wants truth, appreciation and acknowledgement. The same dignities you'd afford someone else, could be allowed to be spent on your own being. What is the guilt, shame, embarrassment, fear, annoyance, anxiety or stress that you associate with this is what must be dealt with and overcome in order for you to feel better. So how does one slay this dragon? *You don't.* You let the dragon exist independently of your being and start identifying with something else. Use conscious attention and intention.

BJJ isn't just physical; its therapeutic. It's a healing art and a mental reset. The focus required in BJJ can act as a form of meditation, clearing emotional clutter. Gentle rolling and specific exercises can help rehabilitate injuries. The camaraderie in BJJ provides uplifting during the most needed moments and a sense of belonging.

How you move means something:

Posture will make or break you. Hunching, placing your hips out of alignment with your shoulders and having a weak pelvic floor all contribute to a heaping pile of humanness.

The body is meant to move freely and with ease. If you're creaking and groaning through life that's your sign your body would prefer different ultimately leading to better.

How you talk to yourself:

I'm falling apart

I've got a long road ahead

It's part of getting older

Or

I bounce back like a cat

Clear skies ahead

I'm happy, the best is yet to come!

Say only one set of these three things to yourself for one week all day, everyday. As the only thinker in your head you are the only one with this power.

To approach illness or injury like a warrior let us first understand who it is we're doing battle with. It's not the ailment you face but your relationship to it that is causing you grief.

If you manifested this, it was meant to happen and as it should be. With this acceptance, you can own your reality and your world will be a happier place. Why? Because you deem it as such. By taking control of the narrative you can determine the end of the script. The language used is spoken in cyclical terms by Mother Nature like the golden ratio.

Acceptance sounds like this:

Ex. "My neck injury forced me to chill, spend some time with my loved ones, strategize, get regular massages and start a stretching routine. I'm grateful for all these things in my life and it's only going to get better. Things are turning out really well for me."

Linear rational thinking of the mind sounds like this:

Ex. "My neck is bullshit. This sucks so bad! I'm missing tons of training and still have to pay! Of course I tore up my whole back now, I should have went harder. Now I'll have to quit. My life blows."

Put simply, you can step on a stone (a stepping stone that gains you leverage and a different viewpoint) or beat yourself with it.

You can be in pain without suffering. You cannot be in suffering without pain.

Affirm this to yourself. "I choose my attitude about _____." Remember to pick the voice of your inner warrior, the one who fights till the end for your ultimate best. Either way, you can at least start to appreciate with awareness who is condemning or consoling you.

Example

You're asked by a training partner:

"Hey, how's the knee?"

Pause. Breathe. This is your moment to seal your fate, to write your destiny, choose wisely. . .

In one version of reality you will set the scene for non stop chaos.

Imagine one version of you saying:

"It's the worst, my knee is awful! Training is shit and I'm never finding time to make it in anyway. But what can I do? I'm getting old and the Doctor said there's nothing I can do to fix it."

Now imagine how this version of you will answer the same question three months later:

"I had surgery on my busted knee. It was brutal! I can't do anything I used to and am getting no sleep. It's getting worse and My doctor says I'll need another surgery."

Now let us approach the same question but use our imagination to create a different answer and see if we can feel our way through the outcome.

"Hey, good to see you. I'm here soaking up the good vibes for now. I'll be ready to roll soon, so for now I'm working on some of the modifications and physical therapy stuff."

Based on that answer what would the future hold for this individual? Probably something along the lines of "I'm feeling great. My knee is doing better. I've been working on my bottom side mount so watch out for my new moves!"

Mind heart unity will heal the physical body through appropriate action.

Nurse your whole self. Thoughts. Breath. Action.

Your world will reflect this healthy lifestyle. Being a mentor and form of inspiration will be an everyday occurrence just by leading your life. This is how you contribute to your society and community.

It begins and ends with you. Stay laser point focused on your healing and feeling great as you put your blinders on to anything or anyone less than this goal. You will be granted your wish so it's **best to know what you**'re asking for.

There is not one universal recipe for recovery.

Ask yourself:

Where am I putting my attention?

What am I willing to limit, let go off that is not of my highest good?

Who do you think you are? If you see yourself as a person of value who's wellbeing has worth versus a nobody your treatment will be just that.

Define illness then put it in the mold of a human being. What would that think, speak, act and look like?

How am I being of service? How often am I assisting with my own self and what is the kind and quality of care I am giving to me?

If I lived with this the rest of my life three ways I would control it:

Example: Knee surgery

1. Injury prevention with a knee brace and recovery through heat therapy with a magnesium bath

2. Replace De La Riva with Spider Guard, pick partners, include hip opening warm up stretches and cool down

3. Limit who I grapple with and don't use that side leg

How do I get to do the things I want to do?

Do I have an active or passive approach to healing? Do I want to let someone else take the wheel or take ultimate authority and make use of what I've got?

Just like you'd see an armbar like a movie in your head you can play your character healing and being fully recovered in your mind. What would you allow your movie to look like?

Let's pretend it is me who is hurt and you the reader are now providing me with your experience and knowledge. What could you teach me? What would you intentionally leave out because it wouldn't be helpful? What's your sage wisdom?

Betterments:

- Health = happiness. Doing saying / acting / being in love
- Well-being = following your path of highest good based on something grander than yourself
- Recovery = Let the body speak then honor how you may be of service to to your healing
- Healing = Your attention to wellness and ease

General Tips, Tricks and Hacks:

Work surrounding muscles. Work the complete opposite end.

Do Less. No matter how great you're feeling in the moment go around 20% less (speed, strength, etc.) than you would normally go at your level to ensure a great time without having to compromise your tomorrow.

It's alright to give it time. Tell yourself this instruction daily with kind authority. But remember, this isn't an excuse to check out of training. Secure your fate in other forms like strength training a certain area or grappling related cardio.

Strategize your next moves. Get the rest of your life right squared away so everyone in it can help support you in maintaining your regimen.

Take charge of whatever manifests and responsibility for your perception of it as a positive thing in your life.

A bird has a nest. A beaver has a dam. Has a structure been imprisoned on you? No competition = no belt, Not rolling with everyone = no stripe. You can update what you prescribe to at anytime for immediate relief to any of these symptoms.

Start. If you can't yet play the game. Get game ready. Prepare your body, life and psyche to plan on playing again.

Create a soundtrack to your life. Curate a list to wake up with, work out too and wind down with.

Move your mind. Control your imagination from a friend's point of view.

Notice when you speak what you give your awareness to. Focusing on the pain is literally awful. Allowing your attention to stay connected to feeling the end goal will always guide you in the direction you want to go.

Limit your intake of negativity, violence, sadness, and anything that is going to make you in a worse mood. Call on your Inner Warrior to change the channel.

Try this - LDA

Limitation: Name what you're going through

Definition of: List all you intend to feel different / better

Action: An intention of the steps needed to get you to different

Replacing Jiu-Jitsu with addiction is life saving.

If you've given it all you've got, take.

Take a break

Take your time

Take the first step

Take initiative

Take a load off

Take control

Take back your power

Take it all in

Take a leap of faith

Take a different approach

Take your turn

Alternative Choices

If you perceive a form of treatment as dangerous your ability to react to it is forced through the fight or flight channel. Would it be easier to solve a complex puzzle with a clear mind or a clogged cranium? In this section we look at some of the latest and greatest methods of healing. It's important to do your own research and due diligence before considering anything.

Testosterone Replacement Therapy (TRT) -

The most common, and least often discussed is TRT (testosterone replacement therapy). I will start by saying I don't take TRT and have no personal experience using it. If you're considering it, I would urge you to do intensive research first and talk to your doctor and family members. I will say that as a fifty plus man that TRT is heavily marketed as a "cure-all" for men.

If you're an over 40 competitor you have to be aware that many of your fellow competitors may be using TRT. Since tournaments don't test for it, users aren't doing anything wrong. If someone is using it, there's more than likely a good reason for it. But we can't underplay the fact that they may have a physical advantage compared to their non-TRT counterparts. Some of the reported benefits of TRT are: improved strength and muscle mass, better energy and endurance, faster recovery.

Potential risks: Increased risk of cardiovascular issues, potential prostate issues, long-term dependancy.

CBD (cannabidiol) -

This is a compound found in the cannabis plant. It's not THC, so it won't get you high. It has become wildly popular in the past several years. Especially in the BJJ world. There are very few long-term studies done on it's therapeutic effects. So you do have to base your research mostly on the reports of others.

There are many potential positive effects for the use of CBD. However, its probably not the cure-all it's been marketed to be. It is considered safe, but you do want to make sure it comes from a reputable high quality source.

Potential benefits - Can hep with sleep, recovery / inflammation, possible pain management.

Potential risks - Low quality product (always check the source), may interact with certain medicines, can cause side effects in some people.

Peptides -

These are short chains of amino acids, which are the building blocks for proteins. They are produced by the body and are very important in the process of repairing tissue, inflammation prevention and hormone production. Like TRT, peptide therapy is only diagnosed and performed by a medical professional.

Potential benefits - Pain management, tissue repair and growth, improved sleep, improved immune function.

Potential risks - This is a relatively new field where more research is needed. It is considered controversial and is banned in many professional sports.

Stem Cell Therapy -

Also called regenerative medicine, uses stem cells to help damaged and diseased tissue to heal. It is a field of medical study that is making fast progress and has shown promise in treating a number of diseases and conditions.

Potential benefits - Improved joint health, repaired tissue and regeneration, better recovery and pain management. Has shown potential in slowing age related changes.

Potential risks - While it has shown great promise, it's still being studied and is a relatively new field. It is not regulated by the FDA and costs may not be covered by insurance carriers.

Helping Hands -

Religion, Spirituality and Mindset can greatly impact your path.

Have a mustard seed of faith. A belief in God or higher power can provide some with immense comfort. Trusting may give motivation. Allow hope to inspire action. Belief takes you beyond the ordinary. My belief in a guardian angel has immensely impacted me though my darkest moments. I believe Mike has a connection with Bruce Lee that is beyond this world. Using these perceptions of reality is the lens that combines my heart and mind and I'd recommend it to everyone.

Mission:

Effective recovery is as critical as the training itself. It includes active rest, proper nutrition, and mental relaxation.

Enhance recovery protocols with more advanced techniques and specialized massage therapies.

Implement a personalized recovery plan that includes a mix of physical, nutritional, and mental recovery strategies.

Debriefing Assessment:

Reflect on your current practices for preventing injuries during training and competition. Consider the various components of your injury prevention strategy, such as warm-ups, strength conditioning, technique refinement, and the use of protective gear. Evaluate how effectively these practices mitigate the risk of injury.

Are there areas where you could improve or new tactics you might incorporate into your routine to enhance safety and performance?

Recovery is as vital as the training itself in the life cycle of a BJJ practitioner. Assess your recovery processes, focusing on both immediate post-training recovery and long-term recuperation strategies.

How do you address muscle soreness, manage fatigue, and ensure your body recuperates adequately?

Reflect on the role of sleep, nutrition, hydration, and active recovery techniques like stretching in your recovery regimen.

Consider any recovery aids you use, such as massage therapy or cold and heat treatments, and their effectiveness.

Survival Expert:
MIKE JOLLY

Mike is a former UCLA football player, the inventor of the Iron Neck, and a passionate advocate for concussion prevention. Inspired after seeing the impact concussions had on his former teammates, Jolly's Iron Neck has been widely adopted from youth sports to professional sports leagues across the world.

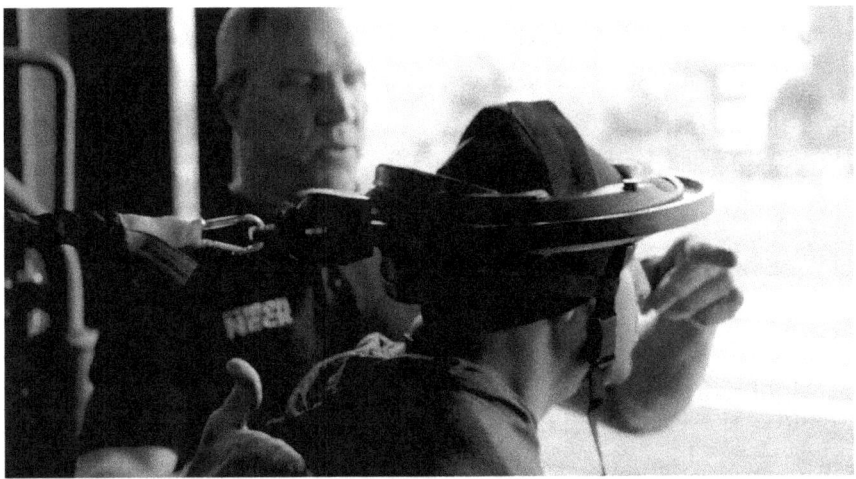

Intel:

I came across Mike Jolly's work with the Iron Neck just a few years ago. I had suffered head and neck trauma many times throughout my martial arts career. Starting from white belt, I was slammed on my neck during competition while trying to execute an armbar. I ended up with a severe concussion, a bulging disk in my neck and long term pain. Over the years I have had additional head trauma from knees, elbows and kicks to the head and face.

In 2017 I was accidentally kicked in the head during a grappling match with a beginner. My partner heel stomped my face causing a fractured nose and a TBI (traumatic brain injury). My head injury left me with constant ringing in my ears (tinnitus), weakness in my neck and back, numbness in my fingers / toes and ongoing headaches. I began researching concussions and learned that they are really caused by a weak neck. The rapid acceleration and deceleration of the brain within the skull causes the injury. Having a weak neck directly impacts the severity of the trauma. Unfortunately there's not a lot of great neck exercises that can be done safely with free weights or body weight.

I was excited when I came across the Iron neck device on an episode of the "Joe Rogan podcast." After a few months using the Iron Neck I was blown away by my results. I was able to restore strength to my neck, shoulders, traps and back. This has resulted in far less time off from the mats due to chronic pain and numbness. I also feel a renewed sense of safety with my grappling. Before I felt compromised whenever someone stacked me up in guard. Now I can train with confidence and longevity.

Straight from the Source:

How can older BJJ practitioners strengthen their necks to prevent injury?

Carefully! As I have gotten older it has been difficult to make myself slow down and approach exercise in a more conservative way. So the first thing I would say is if you haven't been training your neck start slow and ramp up as your neck strength increases. Then the question is how do I train the neck effectively and safely?

What's the best way to deal with chronic neck pain that results from practicing BJJ?

If a practitioner has chronic pain he should turn to a medical professional to make sure that structurally it is safe to continue training. If the answer is yes then the athlete must strengthen the neck, increase flexibility of the neck and increase range of motion of the neck. These are the three keys to getting rid of chronic pain. I have seen miraculous recoveries with fighter pilots. During the install and orientation of Iron Necks at Luke Air Force Base I met several veteran pilots who had the most damaged necks I have ever seen. Iron Neck, along with trainers pushing the pilots to train, reduced the chronic pain to negligible levels. Point is it works - by building neck strength safely and methodically, increasing ROM (range of motion) and flexibility we can become pain free.

How can older BJJ practitioners balance the demands of training with the need to keep their necks healthy?

We have so many demands on our time it is hard to fit in everything we want to do. Here's the bottom line - BJJ practitioners can't afford to not to train their necks. The good news is training with the Iron Neck is very efficient. The six foundational exercises take less than six minutes to complete. That is a small sacrifice to reduce chronic pain and prevent future injuries. Here is an example of what six minutes three times a week can achieve: We had high school football coaches keep records of the gains their athletes made in neck size on a month by month basis when they instigated the training protocol. On average the athletes put on two inches of circumference in two months. That is a lot of injury preventing muscle in a short period of time.

What is your general advice for practitioners over 40 who want to keep their necks healthy while continuing to enjoy BJJ?

Strengthen it. Obviously the neck is an integral part of BJJ. Where the head goes the body follows. You can't let anyone control your head, and the only way to prevent someone from controlling your head is by having a very strong, flexible neck that can withstand the forces being applied. You certainly can't enjoy BJJ with a weak neck that allows you to be controlled, or a neck with chronic pain, or a neck with limited range of motion. You must train your neck and train it to resist the violence experienced in a match if you want to keep enjoying BJJ after 40.

Can you recommend any post-training recovery techniques specifically aimed at reducing neck strain or tension?

A great massage, Thera-Gun, a hot spa with strong jets have always been my go to. In addition to injury prevention benefits of Iron Neck, it is also an incredible mobility maker. Lighter band tension and a greater focus on fluid movements with Iron Neck post-training is a great addition to the protocol.

What role does mental preparedness play in preventing neck injuries in BJJ, especially for older practitioners?

To be mentally prepared you have to put in the work - and a large part of that work is physical. If you were a college football coach you wouldn't just keep your team in a classroom all week teaching and quizzing them on their assignments for each play and then send them out to play on Saturday. To be mentally prepared you have to know that you have physically prepared yourself to the best of your abilities.

Here is an example: Aaron Pico was a great wrestler in high school before he became a great MMA fighter. He started training with the Iron Neck when he was 15 years old. I went back to check on him and see how he was progressing after he had been training with the Iron Neck for three months. When he saw me come into the facility he slowly walked over to me, head tipped forward and chin tucked as he looked up at me and said in a very intimidating voice, "Mike, my head is now a weapon." Do you think Aaron was mentally prepared? He knew no one was going to control his head and that he would use it to control them. He won four State of California titles.

You will have a less likely chance of getting injured if you have put in the work and know you are prepared. You will fight your fight and not be timid knowing that your neck is a strength not a weakness.

The Role of Jiu-Jitsu in Personal Development

This art molds the mind, body, and spirit. As practitioners, we often focus on the physical aspects of training, but the true power of Jiu-Jitsu lies in its profound impact on personal development. The discipline, challenges, and community inherent in BJJ foster significant growth, resilience, and a relentlessly positive mindset.

At its core, BJJ requires a deep commitment—a discipline that extends far beyond the mats. The routine of regular practice, the dedication to improving techniques, and the persistence in facing and overcoming challenges are all crucial elements that enhance personal growth. This discipline teaches us about setting goals, the importance of consistency, and the value of hard work, lessons that are invaluable in every area of life.

Challenges push you out of your comfort zone, forcing you to adapt and overcome. It's in these moments of struggle that true personal development occurs. We learn to embrace failure as an opportunity to learn, fostering a growth mindset that views setbacks as essential steps in the journey of improvement.

The BJJ community plays a pivotal role in personal development. This community is not just about training partners; it's about forming a supportive network that uplifts each member. From cheering for one another during competitions to providing advice off the mats, the bonds formed are instrumental in fostering a sense of belonging and mutual growth. Learning to give and receive support builds empathy, strengthens social connections, and enhances our emotional resilience.

BJJ not only strengthens the body but also the mind. The regular practice of Jiu-Jitsu can be a powerful tool for managing stress, anxiety, and depression, promoting an overall positive mindset. The focus required on the mats helps clear the mind of external worries, allowing practitioners to return to their daily lives refreshed and with a healthier, more balanced perspective.

Mission:

Through discipline, challenge, community support, and mental fortitude, Brazilian Jiu-Jitsu offers a unique platform for personal development. As we navigate the ups and downs of training, we discover that the lessons learned in Jiu-Jitsu are applicable far beyond the confines of the gym. Embrace this journey with an open heart and mind, and let Jiu-Jitsu shape you into not only a better fighter but a stronger, more resilient individual.

Survival Expert:
MARK 'FUNK' ROBERTS

---

54 years old, online Fitness Expert Entrepreneur
Former Professional Beach and
Indoor Volleyball Player for Canada
Fought professional Muay Thai in Thailand in his 40s.

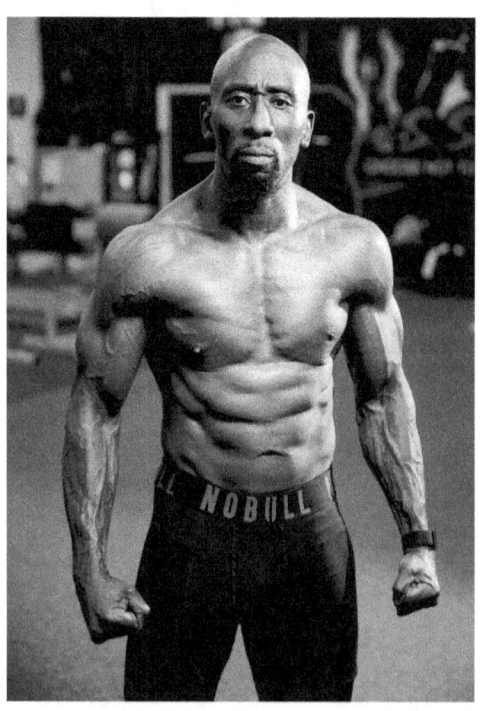

Intel:

Funk currently works with UFC Canada, Australia and New Zealand in Athletes and Fighter Relations and writes articles for MMA, BJJ and Muay Thai magazines, online fitness websites and is part of the Onnit Academy.

With 25 plus years' experience, he has helped millions reach their fitness goals and improve athletic performance through his over 100 online metabolic workout programs. Funk is also a Certified Master Metabolic Trainer, Certified MMA Conditioning Coach (MMACA) NESTA, Certified Fitness Nutrition Coach, Core Conditioning Specialist - NESTA, Kettlebell Training Specialist, Pain-Free Performance Specialist and Mindset Coach.

When Funk turned 40 years old, he struggled with having low testosterone, being overweight and having a puffy, pudge muscle look. After a ton of research, trial and error and putting it into action, Funk has developed a training and lifestyle system for men over the age of 40 who want to get into the best shape of their life.

In 2010, Funk transformed his own body from a puffy 215 lbs to 185 lbs lean ripped and over the past 10 years has been able to naturally maintain his body, health, and youthfulness.

From the Source:

Exercise and fitness is a constant source of inspiration for me. Having experienced firsthand the importance of health and fitness, especially as I aged beyond 40, I have always prioritized it.

My journey as a former professional athlete and Muay Thai fighter has ingrained in me an understanding that one must not only train hard but also smart. You need to balance intensive workouts with sufficient recovery routines to ensure your body remains at its peak.

For me, maintaining a regular workout routine of 4 days a week, coupled with 2 days of recovery, is more than a choice—it's a value system that I've set for myself. It's an essential, non-negotiable part of my life.

Excuses don't have a place here; I either make time for my health and fitness or I make excuses, and I've chosen to always prioritize the former.

Since turning 40, my commitment to maintaining health in all areas of my life has only strengthened. As I've grown older, I've realized that our bodies demand more respect, more care, and more attention. And so, I've made it my mission to not just live this life, but also inspire and guide others to do the same.

For those seeking to stay motivated, my advice is simple but potent:

before you begin, find a strong "WHY".

This "why" is your personal reason for committing to a fitness routine. It could be anything from wanting to feel better about yourself, being around to see your grandkids grow up, or simply keeping up with your daily activities without feeling worn out.

This "WHY" is more than just a goal—it's the fuel that will keep your motivation burning even when the going gets tough. It's what gets you up in the morning for that workout when you'd rather stay in bed. It's the driving force that helps you push through when you feel like giving up.

Remember, your "WHY" is unique to you, and it's one of the most powerful tools you have to stay inspired and motivated on your fitness journey. But you have to dig deep... in other words your "WHY" should make you "CRY!"

It's not just about starting this journey, it's about staying on it, and your "why" is the compass that will keep you on track.

Fitness past Forty:

As we age, our physical capacities, motivations, and lifestyles inevitably change. This impacts the way we approach fitness, and for those of you engaged in Brazilian Jiu-Jitsu, the changes can be even more specific and noticeable.

Let's discuss this in terms of physiology, psychology, and lifestyle:

Physiologically, our bodies go through natural changes as we age. For instance, sarcopenia - the loss of muscle mass due to aging - can kick in.

From our 30's onwards, we also experience a decrease in testosterone levels at a rate of approximately 1-2% per year. This decline directly impacts muscle growth, recovery, and overall physical strength and energy. Coupled with testosterone decrease, our metabolism also begins to slow down. This is often attributed to lifestyle changes such as dietary habits and decreased physical activity.

The implications for fitness are significant: maintaining muscle mass, burning fat, and staying energized becomes more challenging. Furthermore, as we age, our bodies naturally take longer to recover from exercise and injury. This can be exacerbated in a sport like BJJ, which is physically demanding and requires a great deal of resilience. Increased frequency of aches, pains, and injuries due to wear and tear on our joints can also become a factor, adding to the recovery time and affecting consistent training.

Psychologically, our drive and motivation can be influenced by these physical changes. When we constantly have to deal with aches, pains, and longer recovery periods, it can create a mental barrier that wasn't present in our younger years. This shift can be quite challenging to navigate.

Lastly, lifestyle changes as we age play a considerable role. By the time we're in our 40's, many of us have family responsibilities and career demands that take priority. Our time and energy might be more divided, and finding the motivation and room for consistent training can become harder.

Comparatively, when we're in our 20's and 30's, many of these factors aren't as prevalent. High testosterone levels, faster metabolism, quicker recovery times, fewer injuries, and a generally more flexible lifestyle often allow us to train more intensively and regularly. Therefore, when it comes to fitness and particularly BJJ for those over 40, it's important to understand and adapt to these changes.

It's about training smart, focusing on nutrition, prioritizing recovery, and maintaining a strong mental game to navigate the challenges. The journey might look different, but the passion and benefits of BJJ and fitness remain.

Conditioning Catered to Over Forty BJJ:

Brazilian Jiu-Jitsu demands a great deal of physical capacity and conditioning, covering diverse attributes like aerobic and anaerobic fitness, overall strength, muscular endurance, mobility, flexibility, core strength, explosive power, speed, and effective fat management.

Here are some exercises and workout types specifically tailored for those over 40 to enhance these areas:

Aerobic Fitness: The focus here is on improving cardiovascular endurance.

Low-Impact Steady State (LISS) cardio: This might include brisk walking, cycling, or swimming for around 30-60 minutes. LISS cardio can help build an aerobic base without causing too much strain on the joints.

Rowing: If you have access to a rowing machine, this is an excellent full-body cardio workout.

Circuit training: Lightweight and high repetition circuits with short rest periods can significantly improve cardiovascular endurance.

Anaerobic Fitness: This pertains to short, intense exercises that improve power and speed.

Metabolic Bodyweight Workouts:

Using your own bodyweight in workouts is huge for BJJ athletes. Alternating between intense bursts of exercise and fixed periods of less-intense activity or even complete rest. So including metabolic circuits with fundamental movement exercises like:

Lunge variations – for example: reverse, forward and stationary lunges, low lunge, isometric lunges, step ups and jumping lunges

Squat variations – regular squats, cycle squats, staggered squat, wall squats, jump squats

Push variations both horizontal and vertical – push ups variations and dips

Pull variations both horizontal and vertical – pull ups and bodyweight inverted rows

Hip Hinge exercises - bodyweight jumps, hip hinge exercises

Core exercises – side planks, plank variations and more.

Tabata Training: This is a type of HIIT where you work hard for 20 seconds and rest for 10 seconds, repeating this for 4 minutes. Great to use Tabata Burpee Finishers after a BJJ session

Overall Strength and Muscular Endurance:

Resistance Training:

Workouts involving weights or resistance bands are excellent for building overall strength. Dumbbells can be particularly beneficial for enhancing grip strength and engaging stabilizing muscles in the core. Examples of exercises include dumbbell squats, lunges, chest press, shoulder press, bicep curls, and tricep extensions.

Bodyweight Exercises:

Squats, lunges, push-ups, and pull-ups can improve muscular endurance and strength without the need for equipment.

Kettlebell Workouts:

Swings, goblet squats, and Turkish get-ups, farmers walks are great full-body workouts.

Mobility and Flexibility:

- Yoga: Gentle yoga can enhance both flexibility and mobility, key components for BJJ.

- Animal Flow movement patterns are great to help with movement and mobility.

- Dynamic Stretching: Unlike static stretching, dynamic stretching involves movement and can be a great way to improve mobility.

- Foam Rolling: This can help with muscle recovery and improve flexibility.

Core Strength: Certainly, core strength, especially in the context of BJJ, involves a broad range of stability and movement, including anti-rotation, rotation, anti-flexion, extension, core stability, and anti-lateral flexion.

Anti-Rotation:

- Pallof Press: This is performed with a resistance band or cable machine and helps improve your ability to resist rotational forces.

Rotation:

- Medicine Ball Russian Twists: These target rotational muscles and can be modified based on your skill level.

Anti-Flexion & Extension:

- Dead Bugs: This exercise strengthens your core while teaching your body to resist extension.

- Bird Dogs: This exercise helps resist extension and also promotes stability.

Core Stability:

- Stability Ball Planks: These can enhance core stability by introducing an unstable surface.

- Stir the Pot: This is another stability ball exercise that targets the entire core.

Anti-Lateral Flexion:

- Side Planks: These directly target the lateral core, helping prevent lateral flexion.

- Suitcase Carries: Walking with a weight in one hand helps train the body against lateral flexion.

Grip Strength: Grip strength is also crucial in BJJ given the need for strong holds and maneuvers.

- Farmer's Walks: Simply carrying heavy weights for an extended period is a great way to build grip strength.

- Pull-ups / Hang: Not only do these build upper body strength, but maintaining a hold on the bar improves grip strength.

- Wrist Curls and Reverse Wrist Curls: These can be performed with dumbbells to directly target the muscles involved in grip.

Explosive Power and Speed:

- Plyometrics: Exercises like jump squats and burpees can build explosive power.

- Sprinting: Short, intense bursts of running can significantly improve speed.

- Box Jumps: These improve lower body power and speed.

Fat Loss:

- HIIT Workouts: These are great for burning fat due to the high calorie expenditure both during and after the workout.

- Circuit Training: These can be adjusted to be intense and quick, increasing the potential for fat burning.

- Resistance Training: Building more muscle can increase your metabolism, aiding in fat loss.

Remember, the key to effective training, especially as we age, is to listen to your body. Ensure you are getting proper rest and recovery, maintain a healthy diet, and always warm-up before exercising to avoid injury.

Debunk with Funk:

1. "You cannot build muscle after 40"

This is a widespread misconception. While it's true that the body's muscle-building process slows down with age due to factors like decreased testosterone levels, it doesn't mean that muscle building becomes impossible.

With the right resistance or strength training regime and proper nutrition that promotes muscle growth and repair, one can indeed build muscle after 40.

For instance, a metabolic resistance training routine comprising three total body workouts per week can effectively stimulate muscle growth.

Moreover, maintaining a balanced diet rich in protein, healthy fats, and complex carbohydrates is key to muscle repair and growth. It's about consistent effort, smart training, and nutrition, rather than just youth.

2. "You cannot get fit after 40"

Another myth that I'd like to debunk is that achieving fitness after 40 is an unattainable goal. While it's true that the body undergoes physiological changes that might make it slightly more challenging to maintain or achieve peak fitness, it's far from impossible.

However, the margin for error does become smaller.

This means that there needs to be a greater focus on training, sleep, recovery, nutrition, and supplementation.

Fitness after 40 is not just about the intensity of your workouts, but also about the quality of your recovery and nutritional intake. It's about adopting a holistic approach to health and fitness that encompasses all aspects of your lifestyle.

3. "The 'Dad Bod' is great"

The term "Dad Bod" has been popularized and even celebrated in recent years, often referring to a physique characterized by moderate muscularity and increased body fat, especially around the abdomen.

However, despite its seemingly harmless and even endearing connotation, it can potentially mask serious health implications.

Carrying excess subcutaneous fat, especially around the midsection, can lead to increased estrogen levels and decreased testosterone in men.

This hormonal imbalance can negatively impact muscle mass, energy levels, mood, and overall health.

Additionally, increased body fat is associated with a greater risk of chronic health issues such as heart disease, diabetes, and certain cancers.

While it's crucial to promote body positivity and acceptance, it's equally important to be aware of the potential health implications that come with excess body fat.

Fitness and health are about more than just appearances; they're about taking care of your body to lead a long, fulfilling life. Remember, it's never too late to make positive changes towards a healthier lifestyle, regardless of your age.

Frequency and Intensity of Workouts:

To make continued progress in BJJ and overall fitness past the age of 40, it's crucial to take a strategic and holistic approach to planning workout routines.

Here's how to adjust the frequency and intensity of workouts while still seeing improvement:

1. **Identify Your BJJ Training Days:** The first step is to set a consistent schedule for your BJJ sessions. Let's say these are twice a week.

2. **Incorporate Core Training:** Core strength is essential for BJJ and general fitness. You could incorporate core workouts on the same day as your BJJ training, either before or after depending on what works best for you. Exercises that involve anti-rotation, rotation, an-

ti-flexion, extension, core stability, and anti-lateral flexion should be included.

3. **Plan for Conditioning:** Conditioning is a critical aspect of fitness, helping improve stamina, strength, and power, all of which are essential for BJJ. This could also be done after your BJJ sessions or on separate days.

4. **Workout Days:** If you train BJJ twice a week, you might schedule two additional total body workout days. These workouts, around 30-40 minutes, could involve resistance training, cardio, and targeted exercises for areas you want to improve. You could finish each session with a short high-intensity finisher or a core circuit for a well-rounded workout.

5. **Recovery Routines:** Recovery is an often-overlooked aspect of fitness that becomes increasingly important as we age. Dedicate at least two days a week for recovery routines. This could involve practices such as yoga or pilates, which promote flexibility, strength, and mindfulness. Mobility exercises are also essential to maintain a good range of motion and can help with recovery and injury prevention.

6. **Rest Day:** Lastly, don't forget to include at least one full rest day in your weekly schedule. This is a day where you refrain from both BJJ and intense workouts, allowing your body to rest and repair.

The goal here is to train effectively, allowing enough time for recovery, which is paramount in avoiding injury and promoting progress.

This might look like four days of BJJ and workouts, two days of recovery routines, and one full rest day. This structured approach will ensure you maintain a balanced and manageable routine that will facilitate ongoing progress in your fitness and BJJ skills. Remember, consistency is key.

The BJJ Brain:

Mindset plays an incredibly crucial role in staying active and competitive in BJJ, particularly as one ages. It's the foundation upon which all your training, habits, and results are built. Here's why:

Acceptance: With age, physical abilities naturally diminish. Understanding and accepting these changes is the first step. It doesn't mean you can't be competitive or improve; it means your training and recovery might look different from a 20-year-old's.

Acceptance allows you to make the necessary adjustments to your routine without feeling defeated or discouraged.

Resilience: BJJ, like any other competitive sport, will have its challenges, setbacks, and losses. An older athlete's resilience, the ability to bounce back from these challenges, is heavily reliant on mindset. Seeing these as learning opportunities rather than failures encourages continual growth and improvement.

Patience: Progress may be slower as we age due to physiological changes. The ability to be patient with your body and your progress becomes even more critical. Mindset plays a huge role in fostering patience and keeping frustration at bay.

Discipline and Consistency: Staying competitive means consistent training, good nutrition, adequate sleep, and regular recovery routines. The discipline to stick to these habits even when it's difficult is a mental game.

Purpose: Knowing your "why" keeps the fire lit. Why do you train? Why do you compete? Is it for health, the thrill of competition, the camaraderie? Having a strong sense of purpose fuels motivation, particularly during challenging periods.

Positive Self-Talk: As we age, it's easy to fall into the trap of self-limiting beliefs. Engaging in positive self-talk, reminding ourselves of our capabilities and accomplishments, and visualizing success can significantly impact performance and the enjoyment of the sport.

Adaptability: As we age, the ability to adapt our training routine, intensity, and even our BJJ techniques is crucial to avoid injuries and stay competitive. An open mindset that embraces change and adaptation can be a game-changer.

In summary, the physical act of engaging in BJJ is just one part of the equation. A positive, resilient, and adaptable mindset is just as, if not more, important in staying active and competitive as we age.

Staying Strong:

As an athlete ages, especially one involved in a physically demanding sport like BJJ, it becomes imperative to tweak traditional strength training methodologies to better suit their needs. The goal is to maximize results, minimize risk, and promote longevity in the sport. Here's how:

1. **Shift from Maximal Strength to Muscular Endurance:** Traditional powerlifting exercises such as deadlifts, squats, and bench presses focus primarily on maximal strength. While these exercises have their place, the risk-to-reward ratio might not be suitable for athletes over 40, particularly those involved in BJJ. The sport requires not just strength, but muscular endurance - the ability of your muscles to exert force over a sustained period.

2. **Limitations of Traditional Powerlifting:** High-intensity powerlifting workouts (Cross fit) can be quite taxing, leaving less energy for other critical aspects of training. They also have a higher risk of injury, especially if proper form is not maintained, which can be detrimental to an aging athlete. Further, mastering the technique of these

lifts can be time-consuming, and that time might be better invested elsewhere for a BJJ athlete.

3. **Incorporate Kettlebells:** Kettlebell training provides an excellent alternative to traditional powerlifting. Kettlebells are versatile and can be used for a variety of exercises that target strength, muscular endurance, and even cardiorespiratory fitness. Importantly, they also engage the core and promote stability, crucial for BJJ. The movements are generally more natural and less taxing on the joints than heavy powerlifting, making them a safer option.

4. **Functional Training:** Exercises that mimic the movements and challenges faced in a BJJ match can be incredibly beneficial. This could include workouts focusing on grip strength, rotational and anti-rotational core exercises, and movements that enhance agility and speed. Dumbbell training can be particularly effective here, enhancing functional strength and stability.

5. **Consistent Progression:** Whatever the chosen method of strength training, it's essential to have a progression plan. Whether it's increasing the weight of the kettlebell, the number of reps, or the complexity of the movement, progression is key to continued improvement.

6. **Balanced Approach:** Finally, remember that strength training is just one component of fitness for BJJ. Flexibility, cardiovascular fitness, technical skills, and recovery are equally important. A well-rounded fitness program will ensure that you are not just strong, but also durable, agile, and resilient.

The key is to be smart about your strength training.

Choose methods that are going to offer the best benefits for your BJJ and grappling, while minimizing the risk of injury and overtraining.

With age comes wisdom, and part of that wisdom is knowing how to adapt your training to best serve your goals and longevity in the sport

Strength training is important but with so many other physical attributes needed for BJJ and as an aging athlete over 40 you have to be smart with the type of strength training that you do.

Warrior Fuel:

You can't out train a bad diet...Nutrition is a critical factor in maintaining fitness, especially for an athlete over 40. It affects everything from muscle growth and recovery to hormone balance and overall health. Here's how to best fuel your over 40 body:

Balanced Meals: Aim for at least three meals a day, each consisting of a good balance of macronutrients. Include complex carbohydrates like basmati rice, steel cut oats, sweet potatoes, or legumes to provide steady energy and support muscle and brain health. Carbohydrates also aid in thyroid function, which is crucial for metabolism.

High-quality Protein: Protein is the building block of muscle and is vital for repair and recovery post-training. Choose high-quality sources like lean meats, fish, eggs, or legumes. Adequate protein intake helps to maintain muscle mass and aids in hormone regulation, which is essential for overall health and performance.

Healthy Fats: Foods rich in healthy fats like avocados, olive oil, nuts, seeds, and fatty fish provide necessary cholesterol, which is a precursor for testosterone production. Testosterone is crucial for muscle development and overall vitality.

Fruits and Vegetables: Rich in antioxidants and other micronutrients, fruits and vegetables support overall health, immune function, and recovery. They also provide dietary fiber, which is important for digestion and satiety.

Nutrient Timing: Consuming slow-digesting carbs before training, like a pear or whole grain bread, can provide sustained energy. A post-training meal should ideally have a 3:1 carb-to-protein ratio to replenish glycogen stores, aiding in recovery and preparing your body for the next workout.

Hydration: Aim for at least a gallon of water a day, with increased intake on training days. Hydration is vital for optimal bodily function, including nutrient transport, digestion, and temperature regulation.

Supplementation: While a balanced diet should provide most of your nutrient needs, some supplements can offer additional benefits. Creatine can enhance athletic performance by providing energy to your muscles. Omega-3 fatty acids support heart and brain health.

Probiotics aid in digestion, vitamin D3 is crucial for bone health and immune function, and a high-quality multivitamin can fill in any nutritional gaps.

BCAAs (branched-chain amino acids) can aid muscle recovery, and electrolytes help maintain fluid balance, especially during intense training.

Protein Shakes and Testosterone Boosters: Adding a high-quality grass-fed whey protein shake to your day ensures a steady supply of amino acids for muscle repair and growth.

Also, a high-quality testosterone booster can help support hormone balance, particularly for men over 40.

Greens and Beta-Alanine: Greens supplements can help ensure you're getting all the necessary micronutrients, especially if your vegetable intake is less than optimal.

Beta-Alanine is a pre training supplement known to improve muscular endurance, which can be beneficial for BJJ training.

Remember, every individual is different. What works best for one person may not work as well for another.

Operations:
<u>Beyond Black Belt</u>

Post-black belt mastery involves evolving your personal style, exploring new techniques, and embracing teaching. This chapter discusses continuous personal and technical growth, influencing and inspiring future generations.

Scan the QR code for guidance on lifelong training
and evolution beyond the black belt.

https://www.youtube.com/playlist?list=PLwb5iQup993-
QMLj6FcEqr8w024Gb-d6P

BJJ Road Blocks

As 40 plus practitioners we are each unique to ourselves and bring a lifetime of experiences, wear and tear and personal attributes to the mats. Our past experiences can both support and sometimes hinder our progression. Below I give a list of twenty possible roadblocks a 40-plus practitioner could face on their journey. With each one I share accompanying solutions and strategies.

"I'm a slow learner" -

Consider taking private lessons. If budget constrains are a concern inquire about privates with an under belt. Videos, books and multi media learning can be helpful. This can include online courses and instructional videos. Just be careful you don't "muddy the waters" by over stimulating your BJJ brain.

"I have no cardio or stamina" -

Sometimes we can be tricked into thinking a better gas tank is the answer. I would go back to mastering your technique first and foremost. Are you moving efficiently or wasting energy? A grappling match is not just a marathon, it's also a sprint. But you have to know when to utilize each one. Build your BJJ IQ, but with a solid cardio baseline.

"I am extremely inflexible" -

You don't need to do the splits to practice BJJ. In fact the most effective techniques don't require you to be flexible at all. But adding flexibility to your game can prevent injuries and make training more fun. Having some pliability does allow you to do more. But it's certainly not a necessity. However that doesn't mean you shouldn't stretch! Invest time into your flexibility. Spend 15-20 minutes per day mindfully stretching. Throw on your ear phones and a nice piece of music and your body will thank you the entire time!

"I have too many commitments" -

Everyone has a busy life. Yet somehow people make it to black belt in BJJ. *Review what we discussed in the chapter on time management. Be creative with your time and schedule. You can look into private lessons as an option. Most instructors can do them at off times that can accommodate a busy schedule. Remember, everyone needs an outlet. Something to "plug into" and let off the steam. Your BJJ training is important to every part of your life!

"I cannot pay for tuition" -

Be honest and open and discuss your situation with your professor. You can offer to trade for lessons (cleaning, painting, skill trade, assisting in kids classes, etc.) Online courses can also be a temporary solution.

"I'm always injured" -

Ask yourself why? Are you training too hard or too often? Are you in your best physical condition (diet, supplements, stretching, recovery program, etc.) Are you and your partners training safely? Are you having ego flares?

Make whatever modifications are necessary for a safe experience. Keep it sustainable.

"My recovery is too slow" -

First look at your rest, diet, and supplementation. Do you have your "house in order?" Or could you use a little improvement in these areas. Aim for 7-9 hours of sleep every night. Sleep is where your most important recovery work happens. Avoid computers, tablets and phones in bed. If you need noise, turn down the screen and listen as you fall asleep. Try our sleep BJJ meditations too!

"I'm too old and got started to late" -

You're never too old to get started. Look for inspiration from within the BJJ community for others that are your age or older. Discuss with your professor whatever modifications you need for a safe, enjoyable experience. You may consider private lessons as a supplementation to regular group classes.

"There's no school in my city" -

Start one! Maybe you can't open a school, but you can buy mats and put them in your garage or basement. You may be able to find others in your same area who are also interested in learning BJJ. You can create a meet-up for training. You can also travel to nearby towns or cities that may have established programs. When I started BJJ in 1996 I had to travel several hours to train with a black belt. I would go and learn what I could, then travel back and train and share what I learned with my small group. There's also plenty of online courses and video tutorials for additional resources.

"It's mentally too tough for me" -

Start a daily mindfulness and meditation practice. By sitting with your thoughts you can begin to understand yourself on a deeper, more intimate level. If you're just getting started on your BJJ journey, know that it's okay to not know anything and accept that nobody is good right away. Be kind to yourself. If you're more experienced, look how far you've come. It's okay if you still have a ways to go. That's the fun part. "The biggest room in the house, is the one for improvement." Meaning, there's always space for personal growth, on and off the mats.

"I am experiencing PTSD or other mental health challenges" -

BJJ practice can be very beneficial for someone experiencing mental health challenges. However, you should always seek the help of a trained mental health professional if you're experiencing challenges. When you begin BJJ always communicate with your coaches and professors any problems you may be experiencing. Mindfulness meditation can be helpful to improve mental clarity and can have a grounding effect. Be sure to listen to our meditations and visualizations regularly.

"My self or my partner are experiencing health challenges" -

You cannot predict the future. But you can create a healthy lifestyle now that may carry you into the future. Your continued study of BJJ can certainly contribute to a healthy lifestyle. BJJ is the perfect stress reliever. Focusing on training can help you forget about your worries, and physical exercise releases 'feel good' endorphins. By staying in your best physical form you may inspire your partner to do so as well. It is also worthwhile to invite them to training to join you on your wellness journey. The camaraderie from training can also be a great support tool.

"I'm having a disagreement with another student or teacher" -

Open communication is always the key. Schedule a time to speak with your instructor about the situation. Use calm, clear language and explain exactly how you're feeling. If the situation is unresolvable it may be worth considering switching to a new school. Don't quit BJJ over someone else's unmindfulness.

"I feel like I'm not progressing" -

Everyone feels like this from time to time on their journey. Ask yourself what criteria are you using to measure your progress? Belts and stripes come at their own pace in BJJ. If you're waiting every class for a stripe or high five from your instructor, *then you might be disappointed.* Look for other ways to determine your progression. You can seek feedback from your training partners and teachers. The question isn't, "Where's my stripe?" But rather, "What things can I be doing to improve my BJJ?" It might be worthwhile to schedule a private lesson so you and your professor are on the same page.

"I feel like I'm in a slump" -

Everyone reaches the occasional plateau. You might be training too much and may want to consider scaling back slightly. One less day may give you better recovery and a fresh perspective. "Don't live the same day twice." What I mean is mix up your routine and find new ways to challenge yourself. If you always play a top game, try working from the guard instead. Jiu-Jitsu is a very complicated martial arts with many moving parts and an infinite number of moves. Seek out new learning opportunities from seminars, online courses, private lessons, new positions, new training partners, etc.

"I'm too out of shape to do BJJ" -

Remember the point of you training IS to get into your best shape. The good news is that you can't escape it in the practice of Jiu-Jitsu. BJJ forces you into your best physical health. The physical demands of BJJ will guide you to better health. Don't get in shape first and then start BJJ. If you are extremely out of shape, don't panic. You can do this at your own pace. Express your concerns with your professor and create a plan that supports your challenges and makes the appropriate modifications where they are needed. Work on building a healthy lifestyle that balances diet, sleep and recovery. It won't be easy, but it will be worth it!

"I'm not having fun" -

You want to enjoy your BJJ experience but keeping in mind that it's not always going to be sprinkles and sunshine. The training in Jiu-Jitsu may inspire some blood, sweat and tears. (Hopefully not too much blood) The point is that the path to learning Brazilian Jiu-Jitsu is likely to be hard and difficult, but it will also be rewarding and will ultimately change your life in the best ways possible. You will feel a wide range of feelings and physical sensations, from excitement when you learn a new technique to anger and frustration when a sparring partner submits you. This is an important part of the process. This is where you build resolve, patience and endurance, where you develop not just as a martial artist, but also as a complete person. Remember, it won't be tough forever. Look for the small victories along the way that bring you joy.

"I feel like I have too many physical limitations" -

Don't compare yourself to your younger teammates (or your younger self). Your super power is the wisdom from your life experience. You may feel frustration from not being able to keep up with those around you. But remember, that was never the mission. You didn't start BJJ to beat up on the young bucks. Although that always does sound appealing. But I digress. Enjoy where you're today and know that you will improve your physical attributes. Be sure that you're following all of our advice on supplements, recovery, training schedule, sleep, etc. Leave no stone unturned.

"I have an intense fear of getting injured" -

This can be a very real concern that can cause a mental roadblock when you're training. Nobody wants an injury that could interfere with your personal life. Always listen to your body first and foremost. Don't let your own ego, or someone else's, control your actions. Pushing through the pain is never a good idea. Knowing when to propel forward is important, but knowing when to stop is crucial. Some physical discomfort is normal and to be expected during training, but there is a difference between pain that shows growth and pain that indicates possible harm. Understanding this difference can help you avoid injuries and keep you safe on the mat for the long run. It's okay to say "no thanks" to a partner who makes you feel unsafe. Just don't run from challenges as they are crucial to your growth as a student. When you practice moves, never go to the point of pain. The constant locking of your joints can cause overuse injuries. Instead of aiming for pain, focus on perfecting your form and executing the techniques smoothly and effectively.

"I'm too old to start something new" -

Beginning something new can be daunting at any age. When I started BJJ in 1996 it would've been challenging for anyone over 40, let alone folks in their 60's and 70's and beyond to start BJJ. But a new era is upon us, thanks to the growth of the "BJJ After 40" global community. This was also the impetus of this book! To give everyone a clear cut path with complete support along the way. So, no you're not too old. Study this book and we will keep you at your youngest, healthiest self. Look for fellow BJJ practitioners online who are your age or older for inspiration. Trust me there's plenty!

Mission:

It's better to measure your progress based on the bigger picture and not necessarily the day-to-day experiences. Some days you will come to class and feel unstoppable. While others you will be fighting tooth and nail to survive. Some training days are good while others may seem challenging to gain any momentum. Don't fret, as consistency breeds success. If you base your performance on every time you roll, then look for patterns, not huge victories. You want a consistent attendance with relatively consistent results. Nobody is perfect, so you'll experience both highs and lows on the mats. It's important to look for the small victories while acknowledging where you still need work. You can't hide from your failures in BJJ. But also don't beat yourself up either. Look for opportunities for growth.

Begin to explore and use cognitive load theory in your BJJ practice. This can be extremely beneficial in helping you quickly assimilate new moves into your BJJ arsenal. As a professor, I have found this theory very useful in my own teachings. When you're learning new moves, immediately ask yourself, "what is my intrinsic load with this technique?" In other words, what do I already know about it? You can write this out in your BJJ notebook for any new moves you're working through. Next look for opportunities to allow this move to "germinate." This can include: writing out the four steps, teaching it to someone new, videoing yourself performing the move, etc. Utilize my DTP formula for rapid integration: Demonstrate, Teach, Perform.

Don't hesitate to consider solutions for any potential setbacks you might encounter on your journey. Not everything will always be sprinkles and sunshine. By addressing these issues in the present moment, you will equip yourself with resilience and adaptability, hallmarks of a true warrior.

Write out in your BJJ notebook a list of potential hurdles you might face and solutions. Don't hold back, be open and honest. For example: "I am scared of getting hurt" Solution: "I will properly warm up, only train with safe partners, and tap early on everything" Now get to it!

Survival Expert:
GARRY PARRETT

71 years old Wausaukee, WI
Blue Belt under Arete Martial Arts Academy

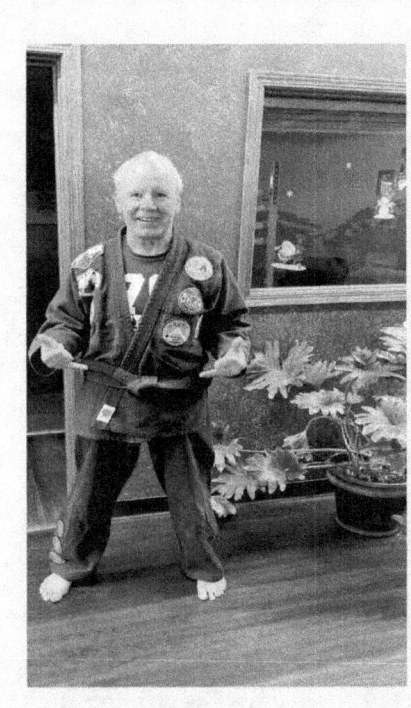
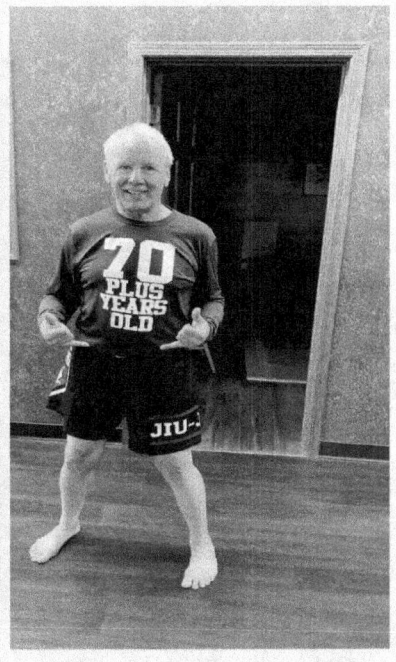

Intel:

I met Garry through the BJJAfter40 private Facebook group. He was hard to miss as he quickly became a "top fan" right away by commenting and posting all the time. He was always very respectful and offered a huge dose of positivity with every interaction.

When I found out he was a 70 year old blue belt I was extremely impressed. It's not like he had been doing BJJ for 40 years and was now 70. He was a longtime martial artist but started BJJ much later in life.

Garry a retired school teacher, is also known as the "Oz Man." He spends his summers running his wildly popular "Wizard of Oz" museum in Wisconsin.

Garry often travels to area open mats and rolls with everyone. Just recently he completed 50 rounds of grappling in just three weeks!

Garry continues to share his spark bringing joy to everyone he interacts with on the mats! Jiu-Jitsu is lucky to have such an inspiration.

Straight from the Source:

I retired from 35 years of teaching (grades 4-8) in 2008.

One day I was driving through a town close to my place where I live. I saw a sign for Tae Kwon do. Since I retired from teaching, I decided to enroll in TKD classes at age 57.

For ten years I trained and during those years I was promoted to third degree black belt. One of the requirements for 2nd and 3rd degrees I had to train in another martial art. I chose ground fighting and Jiu-Jitsu became part of my life for nine years and I'm still at it. I chose two styles : Dan Zan Ryu Jiu-Jitsu (Japanese style) and BJJ. For three years I was doing all three TKD , DZR Jiu-Jitsu and BJJ . After the third year and receiving a purple belt in the Japanese style Jiu-Jitsu, I stopped. I also stopped TKD then too. Since 2014 I have stayed in BJJ and today I still do lessons and travel to roll with younger dudes.

In 2020 I tested for blue and was promoted to the my goal of blue belt just days shy of my 69th birthday.

For almost four years now I do weekly private lessons with my coach. At 70-plus I need these lessons on a one to one basis.

Today I also roll at open mats throughout my home area. I go to five area schools throughout the year. I even drive monthly to a school 100 miles away one way.

I love doing this to represent senior citizens in BJJ and make it known to younger grapplers AGE IS JUST A NUMBER.

I have competed once at a Grappling Industries tournament in 2022 at the age of 70. I did gi and no-gi. I received a 3rd place in no-gi. But my number one win was that I showed up and competed. I am planning one more tournament at 72 years old.

Survival tips from a 71 year old, advice to younger grapplers:

Train weekly at least once

Roll regularly

Train solo drilling techniques at home

Roll at other schools for open mats

Don't give up. Make it fun. Don't let ego dictate your BJJ journey .

Talk to coach regularly. My coach and I talk regularly at my private lessons. He motivates me and teaches what I can do at my age.

I train daily with my Tae Kwon Do and Jiu-Jitsu techniques. I am proud to say that I have done over 4,000 consecutive days since I started solo training.

My unexpected benefits:

I feel young when I come to class and learn and roll.

For me I'm lucky to have no serious injuries.

I am a role model to all ages.

I am more confident in my life.

Younger grapplers are looking up to me… Proud to be rolling with this dinosaur in BJJ.

My coach is number one believer in me. Many times since my blue belt promotion I wanted to retire (another word for QUIT). Jeff Tardiff, my coach and motivator, gives me reasons why I shouldn't. He wants me to stay active physically and mentally. My mom's siblings all had Alzheimer's, luckily my mom at 91 didn't have it. He wants to prevent that in me with doing Jiu-Jitsu. He tests me with reviewing techniques weekly and live rolling with him.

Another motivational factor:

My younger training partners. I feel young when I roll and when they say you are hard to get to submit, that motivates me more with praise. There are two statements while rolling and the rolling partners mentioned these to me :

I can't imagine my Dad or Grandpa doing this.

I hope I can do BJJ at your age.

I always say to new rolling partners don't be easy on me because I won't be to you. I will tap when your technique works on me. I have no ego issues and I want no major injury at anytime.

Creativity in BJJ

The exploration of BJJ offers an infinite number of possibilities. In other martial arts the system is generally based on a small fixed-set of moves. Boxing is made up of four primary offensive moves: the jab, cross, hook and upper-cut. Traditional Karate is made up of seven primary moves: four punches and three kicks (front, side and round house kick). Of course these martial arts offer a far deeper premise when you add additional offensive and defensives movements, blocking, parrying, forms, weapons training, etc.

For practitioners of these traditional arts there is even more depth to be found. The moves themselves can be performed in an unending number of combinations and contexts. Ultimately the techniques never really change or evolve beyond their current form. It is the practitioners themselves who "evolve" them into their own personal style.

But BJJ is a different beast. Jiu-Jitsu delves into a realm of training that seems boundless in its possibilities. Instead of using an offensive framework like boxing or karate. BJJ starts with four primary offensive positions (guard, side control, mount and back). From within these positions you have attacks on all of the limbs from top to bottom (neck, shoulders, elbows, wrists, hips, knees, ankles).

Furthermore you have multiple ways to apply leverage to attack these limbs. Whether it be a strangulation or joint manipulation the opportunities to finish an opponent are endless as you advance in BJJ. To even further complicate it, you have both offense and defensive maneuvers, sweeps and counters! The rabbit hole gets even more vast when you consider variations, innovations, adaptations, sub-positions, gi vs. no-gi and more. On top of all this, BJJ is a living, breathing martial art, always evolving and growing exponentially.

Traditional martial arts are sometimes referred to as "dead arts." This isn't meant as a derogatory statement, but rather an observation of their "preservation-centric nature." Traditional arts, such as Karate or Tae Kwon Do, often emphasize maintaining the purity of the techniques as passed down through generations. The primary focus is on conserving the art's historical integrity, leading to a fixed repertoire of techniques. It isn't the system that evolves, but rather the individual.

In the practice of BJJ there is a "co-evolution" as the art and individual grow together. As practitioners delve deeper into the game of BJJ they often feel the urge to experiment and modify techniques to fit their own body and experience. These adaptations force our partners to evolve with our game. BJJ encourages and almost necessitates constant evolution. When you do one thing, it immediately forces your partner to react in some fashion. This constant interplay of "attack and counter" creates a ripple effect. When you think about it, a single effective change can trigger a cascade of adaptations throughout an entire training group. Imagine that one person starts doing baseball chokes, but the rest of the group isn't aware. He shows up to open mat and slaps and bumps his first partner.

Partner "A" slips in the baseball grips from guard, partner "B" ignores the grips and "passes the guard." As "B" goes to side control, partner "A" turns his hips and sinks in the baseball choke! Partner "B" immediately taps and almost goes to sleep.

Now if he continues this streak on the rest of the group they'll need to adapt or die. I guarantee the next open mat that nobody will just let those grips go in so easily. Now if our baseball choker doesn't adapt to these new changes, then it will be "one hit wonder." The choke would still work but would relegated to a low percentage, high risk "suicide move." You could only pull it out every once in a while and at your own risk.

But let's say he does adapt! For the move to work "A" needs his partner to pass to his right side when he sets his grips. However, if he sets the grips and partner "B" passes to his left the choke won't work. He recognizes this and as "B" goes to his left "A" switches his grips to the other side. This important adaptation completely changes the outcome. Because now he can catch him on either side.

Over time his partners will become even more aware of the baseball choke, so he will be forced to add creativity to the initial set ups. This will further evolve the choke for him and the community around him. But if he stopped at that second open mat when everyone was aware of the choke the development of this particular move within his repertoire would have stalled, and a potential evolution within the community would have been stifled.

This continuous feedback loop of action, counteraction, and adaptation leads to the advancement of the technique. It pushes its boundaries, explores its weaknesses, and uncovers new potential strengths.

It's nearly impossible to "invent" a new move in BJJ. Ben Franklin didn't "invent" electricity, he "discovered" what was already there. Creativity in the art of Jiu-Jitsu can be approached in the same way. We all work from the same palate of "colors." We all have two arms, two legs and a neck. Just as Ben Franklin harnessed a natural phenomena, BJJ practitioners don't really invent new moves. Instead they uncover the myriad of possibilities that exist within the framework of the human body.

I have always been a triangle choker. I'm tall with long limbs so it's probably no surprise to anyone that I would gravitate to leg strangulation techniques. As I developed my triangle attacks I was forced by my training partners to create more intricate attack sequences. The better I got at triangles, the more aware my partners became of my triangle tendencies. This encouraged me to push the envelope in this aspect of my game.

This led me to discover the notorious "Cryangle Choke." Do you know about the Cryangle? It's like the standard triangle choke with an arm inside and the legs wrapped around your neck. However, there's one devastatingly evil addition: your leg is also locked inside! The inclusion of the leg makes this a wickedly uncomfortable position. The trap itself will make you want to tap. But wait there's more… Due the structure of the trap you have access to a strangulation, an armlock and a knee bar off their face!

The inclusion of their leg compromises their base, leaving them with no avenue for escape. Hence the name "cryangle choke" – because it's so intense, you'll feel like crying! Many a good practitioner has shed a tear from this evil submission. For me it was a natural evolution and a move that I would hit from time to time. As I progressed in my cryangle game I came up with more and more entries and set ups.

Initially the move didn't even have a name for me. Until Ione day I laughed out loud and said, "cryangle! that's what I'll call it!" When I eventually put the move on my YouTube channel and other social media outlets it caught a lot of attention. I wasn't that surprised because it had a funny name and was a crazy move. But I wasn't prepared for what the move would truly represent!

These days people know me for my crazy take on Jiu-Jitsu. But just a few years ago almost nobody knew who I was. When I created the online BJJAfter40 community it was after I received my black belt in 2014 (after 13 years at brown belt). I was 45 years old and extremely grateful after being awarded my black belt. With the push for my black also came a host of injuries.

I was in great shape, but physically falling apart. This may sound a bit paradoxical. How could I be fit but injured? Part of the impetus of getting my black belt was my return to competitive BJJ. The training that it required for me to be successful competitor also broke down my body. I felt like I was always injured. Every training session seemed to introduce a new injury, and I often half-jokingly remarked that there wasn't a quadrant of my body that wasn't in pain.

My wife, Sheena (also my co-author for this book), witnessed the toll this took on me firsthand. We've been training partners since she began her BJJ journey 20-plus years ago, and today she proudly wears her black belt that was awarded by me. Watching me grapple with persistent injuries sparked a shared curiosity. Together, we embarked on a mission to delve deep into understanding the intricacies of the human body, seeking ways to optimize performance while minimizing wear and tear.

This quest not only strengthened our relationship, but also gave birth to the BJJAfter40 global community. Initially we only had a handful of followers (which we were always thankful for), but as time grew so did our audience. The online community now connects hundreds of thousands of passionate 40-plus BJJ practitioners throughout the world.

Throughout this journey the ethos for our community has remained the same, "The Best is yet to come." This phrase encapsulates our belief in the unlimited potential of all humans, irrespective of age or past set backs. Initially many of my posts were videos of my performing wild techniques. I felt a need to inspire others through my physical movements and personal expression of Jiu-Jitsu. Some techniques would be more "dialed down" and created specifically for the 40-plus crowd. Whereas other were more technically advanced. The cryangle falls into the latter category.

When I introduced the world to "my creation", some were skeptical while others took it as a personal challenge to hit this crazy move. Some even said it was "impossible" to hit, referring to it as a "unicorn move." I continued to release videos on the cryangle in spite of the varying opinions.

It wouldn't be long before someone did hit one in a pro grappling event in Colorado. I was thrilled to hear the announcer say, "That was a cryangle choke! He just hit a cryangle!" Hearing the weird word I made up being used in the lexicon of BJJ was pretty awesome. Since that first cryangle choke it has been executed in both gi and no-gi events. Including the I.B.J.J.F. Euros, Pan Am's and World championships at the black belt level.

Most recently the cryangle was hit in Mixed Martial Arts by Ahmed "the wolverine" Mujtaba in One Championships. As much as the Cryangle has become my baby, I wasn't her true momma. The move itself has been around for a long time. Some called it the "leg-in triangle" (a boring name by the way).

What I brought to the table was a renewed spotlight on this overlooked technique. I rebranded it, giving it a cool name like "Cryangle" that captures the intense discomfort it inflicts on its recipient. Beyond just renaming it, I delved deeper into its mechanics, refining its application and broadening its scope. Under my guidance, the cryangle has transformed from a niche maneuver into a versatile and widely-recognized technique. However, the real credit goes to members of the BJJ community who have further popularized and expanded the move's potential.

Witnessing the "wolverine" hit this move in his MMA fight in "One Championships" was nothing short of exhilarating. For me it was full circle to see my "brainchild" being perfectly executed under the most intense and hostile conditions of a professional Mixed Martial Arts competition.

After the event I received a very kind voice message from one of his old coaches thanking me for putting the cryangle videos out many years ago.

Such acknowledgment is more than just personal validation; it underscores the impact and reach of the BJJAfter40 community. It reaffirms that our collective efforts are not just about techniques and submissions but about forging connections, spreading knowledge, and influencing the broader martial arts landscape in meaningful ways. To me this was a true collaboration.

Jiu-Jitsu gives us all the free-will and ability to create. The only barriers are the ones we create. As a side note: I have a full length instructional course available on BJJ Fanatics called, "Cryangles, Triangles and Leg Locks!" It covers all the details and intricacies of this exciting technique.

Here are strategies for adding more creativity to you BJJ practice:

Flow paced rolling -

Find a partner who can maintain much slower rolling speed. By adding constraints on the velocity at which you both partners perform, you will find more opportunities for creativity. It's vital to keep your physical speed and strength to about 20-30% effort. By using as little speed and power as possible you will focus more on the proper execution of the technique. Remember by developing our 'technique' we invoke the 'art' in Jiu-Jitsu.

We hear the word "technique" being used so frequently in BJJ. "Use better technique!" can often be heard echoing through a dojo. Your professor may have even given you that advice? But you may be left wondering what does that even mean? What is 'technique'?

It encompasses a sequence of four steps, executed with precision, to achieve a desired outcome. This involves proper weight distribution and leveraging your own body mechanics against your partner's vulnerabilities. When all of this comes into alignment you achieve a successful sweep or submission. This is what I often call, "the magic of Jiu-Jitsu!" But there's really nothing magical about it. It's really the execution of the technology of Jiu-Jitsu that creates the wonder and awe.

If you look at the origin of the word "technology" it comes from two Greek words, "Techne" (art or craft) and "Logia" (meaning study or craft). The word "technique" is also derived from the French word, "Techne" (art or skill). This means the definition of technique could be, "the study of art." So what does all this wordplay mean? In the context of BJJ it helps us to better understand it when a coach yells, "use better technique!" What they're really saying is, "use better art."

Now stay with me. The phrase, 'martial arts' means, "art of war" or "the way of the warrior." As a 40-plus practitioner I have to ask you, do you really need more war? (You'll get plenty of it from the twenty-something year old purple belts) But you'll never beat them with "more-war." By the way, that's the surest path to an injury. You will however overcome it with self-control, finesse and great technique. (Something the young lions won't necessarily have) This is the art of Jiu-Jitsu at it's finest.

Conserve your energy and only use controlled aggression. Being completely passive isn't going to advance your game. Also being overly aggressive will only lead to injury for yourself and your training partners. There is a balancing act that must be adhered to. Measured assertiveness can help you to focus energy into movements when it is needed most. **Good BJJ isn't the absence of aggression, but rather the judicious use of it.**

Flow-paced rolling will open up opportunities you might normally miss grappling at full speed. The difference between the two is like comparing a scenic Sunday drive with an Indy-500 race! The leisurely Sunday drive allows you to experience all of the intricacies and nuances of the moment. You feel the placement of your grips and small shifts in body-weight as you move with, and not against your partner. This mindful approach allows you to experience all of your senses as you grapple.

Going full speed is akin to a high speed, blur of the moment, Indy-500 race. Everything is super intense and requires spilt-second decisions. This rapid-fire style of rolling focuses more on reaction and less on reflection. While there's undoubtedly a "rush" to this style, the details however fall to the wayside. This is great for a cardio-session, but not so great for developing solid, reliable technique.

I would also recommend **videoing these sessions** whenever possible for later reflection and analysis. I have personally discovered more transitions and moves when I do my video analysis than when I was actually rolling. With video review you'll be able to pause, rewind and analyze movements frame by frame. You'll discover your preferences, dissect your mistakes and identify patterns in your game.

Having visual feedback can align theoretical aspects of your game with what actually happens in real-time. For example, you may think that things unravel a certain way in your mind, but in actuality it could be very different. When I show a move often times I will demonstrate to my students what happens when "I actually roll" with it.

I could be teaching an armbar from the mount for example. I'll mount an upper belt and ask them to defend the armbar as I'm attempting to do it. They will often counter my initial move which will lead to small adjustments on my part to successfully execute the armbar. This helps bridge the gap between "ideal" move and "real" world application.

When you use video analysis you have the opportunity to glimpse into your own decision making process during live or flow rolls. With both scenarios you'll have plenty to discover about yourself. But not just where you went wrong, but also what you're doing right. These moments of validation can boost your confidence and let you know you're on the right track with certain techniques. There's great power in bridging theory with real-time practice.

Another great strategy for developing creativity in BJJ is what I call "**restricted rolling.**" With this methodology you create limitations around what you and your partner can and cannot do. Let's say for example you want to learn how to utilize the "lapel" (bottom tail) of your gi as a tool and weapon.

You could grab your bottom right lapel with your right hand and maintain the grip throughout the grappling session. You could add the stipulation that you can't let go of it, but you are allowed to wrap it around your partner's limbs or pass it to your other hand. Even without knowing the technical aspects of its use, you would quickly adapt it to your needs. If you do this enough times you would rapidly develop strategies to fit your demands.

Even with no actual instruction you could very quickly become a "lapel expert." I would recommend that instead of trying to learn a few lapel moves on YouTube, you follow this method. Rather than having a few moves for specific scenarios, you'll develop a deep understanding and intuition around the lapel. This approach will connect you organically to the gi tail allowing it to eventually become an extension of your limb.

We have been talking about the "lapel" here, but really you can approach any technique in Jiu-Jitsu in this manner. People that train with me know me for my triangle choke game. I'm no expert, but it's the most "dangerous" part of my BJJ. Not surprising since I'm physically tall and lanky. But you might be surprised to learn that nobody ever taught me a "triangle based" game of Jiu-Jitsu. ***Everything I have collected is through experience and experimentation.*** I have taken on the "teach a man to fish" mentality. If you truly understand things one way, you understand them in all-ways (always).

I can hit a triangle choke from virtually any position and some that aren't even "real" positions. This collection of attacks and counters came through a patchwork of success and failure. With every mistake and victory my triangle game evolved and got better. It's important to note that guidance from a seasoned black belt is invaluable, there's also immense value in self-discovery and crafting techniques that align with your own approach to Jiu-Jitsu.

Remember Jiu-Jitsu is a game to be played, have fun playing the game. With restricted rolling the possibilities are endless. Here's some possible scenarios that can be utilized to encourage creativity.

No arms rolling -

Tuck your hands into your belt or hold them at your side for no-gi grappling. This will force to use your legs more often. In addition you'll have to find leverage in a whole new way.

Eyes closed grappling -

This is exactly what it sounds like. By closing your eyes your other senses will become heightened. This will allow you to "see more." You'll also build your proprioception or limb awareness (often called the "six sense"). This is like the ability of touching your index finger to your nose with your eyes closed and know where your hand is in space and time.

Positional grappling -

In this drill you will start from non-dominant positions to build escape strategies. For example, you might have your partner start in mount and your job is to escape and achieve a better position. You can also start from non-dominant positions and continue the roll once you escape. Try to find new avenues of escape while not leaning on your normal patterns. This builds resilience, adaptability, and broadens your understanding of positional dynamics. By putting yourself in unfamiliar territory, you're essentially forcing your brain to think outside its normal box. *Remember, creativity thrives in the face of adversity.*

Non-dominant side rolling, drilling and attacking -

If you look closely at your game of Jiu-Jitsu you may notice that you almost always pass the guard on the same side. In fact you might even see that you prefer side control on one side too. This is extremely common as BJJ is taught as a right-handed martial art. Most guard passing for example are generally taught with the passer leading with their right leg and passing to their partners right side (your left side when you're facing them).

The main reason you lead with the right leg is that you need to move your legs in a crossing pattern to pass the guard (one leg stepping in front of the other). If you were to pass to your left but lead with your left leg (non-crossing pattern), it would be easy for your opponent to defend by simply shrimping their right leg through and re-guarding you. Conversely if you passed to your right side you would need to lead with your left leg. Whenever the opposite leg comes across during the guard pass this becomes more difficult to defend.

Why is all this important? The point is that you probably follow more patterns in your training than you suspect. With this drill the goal is to break all of your normal tendencies and find new opportunities. Also by getting familiar with your opposing side you expand your game exponentially. Since everyone tends to follow the same patterns, your partners will not be equally good at defending their non-dominant side. If you're right handed, you'll be weaker at defending an armbar on your left side. You'll also be slower and your timing won't be the same as with your right arm.

The question arises from time to time, when I'm teaching about drilling both sides of the body. Students always ask, "Should I be good at both sides?" The answer is yes and no. With fundamentals I think it makes sense to be good at both sides. But it would be impossible to gain mastery at every part of your BJJ game on opposing sides. This it especially true for a practitioner who may train 2-3 times per week. There's just too many moves and not enough time.

Think about it pragmatically. If you have 100 repetitions of an armbar to complete. You would either have to do 200 to hit both sides or do 50 on each side just to hit the baseline. Either way you would be stretching your efforts thin. While it may seem more advantageous to be bilateral (competent on both sides), the reality is that your body has hard-wired tendencies toward one side. This is why people are either right handed or left handed and almost never ambidextrous. (85 - 90% of the population is right handed, 10-15% is left handed, and less than 1% are mixed handedness) Trying to teach yourself to have mastery on both sides is a fools errand. The only caveat would be when it's your "A-game." For me triangle chokes are my main weapon therefore it made sense to develop both sides. If you love omoplata's for example it would be logical to have entries and attacks on both sides.

Here's a great strategy that will throw everyone off! *Start passing guard to your right side (leading with your left leg).* Most people rarely pass on this side therefore your opponents will be taken by surprise. By doing something unexpected, you exploit their ingrained habits and predictive behaviors. In addition, their defense on the non-dominant side will be slower and weaker. Once you establish side control, your partners will also be weaker at defending and escaping too.

I call this area the "**dark side of the moon.**" I refer to it this way because for most practitioners it's uncharted territory. I've even seen blue and purple belts who reverse their grips and legs when they first end up in 100-kilos (side control) on the opposite side (partners left side). Often times they'll mistakingly tuck their right knee to the head and extend their left leg back for 100-kilos. This of course is backwards but would be correct if they were on their "normal" side.

But due to a combination of old muscle memory and being in a new place they get confused. But with some drilling and practice you could become very proficient on the dark side of the moon. This would open up a whole new world for you that would become a nightmare for your training partners. I cover this topic exclusively in my BJJ Fanatics course entitled: "BJJAfter40: Best Practices."

Lottery of moves -

This is a fun way to explore different techniques. This can be done with a training partner, or in a group environment. Write out techniques on small pieces of paper and put them into a hat (raffle drawing style). For example: You could write submissions like, armbar, rear naked choke, etc. Or it could be specific sweeps, positions, etc. The objective is to draw a technique from the hat (without sharing your move with anyone) and then achieve that technique, whether it's a position, sweep, or submission, during your round of grappling. The real value is in attempting techniques that may be outside of your normal repertoire.

Takedown recovery -

The goal here is to recover safely from successful takedowns. You can start from your feet and have your partner attempt takedowns on you. The objective here would be to offer some resistance but the key would be to let them eventually execute the takedown. Your immediate goal is to recover guard and start the round from there. This not only bolsters your takedown awareness, but also builds resilience and your self-confidence knowing that you can survive takedowns.

Sweep counters -

With this drill you will start from guard, half guard, etc. You will offer some resistance and eventually your partner will sweep you. Your job is to defend the sweep as it's happening. If there's four steps in every technique, you will let them get to step 3-4, before defending the sweep. For example, they may be doing a scissor sweep from guard. As they execute the scissor motion and you're falling, you will immediately shift your hips and recover to the top position. This will help familiarize you with the set ups, dynamics, weight distribution, etc. on various sweeps.

Start from a submission -

*Due to the obvious dangers of submission techniques, you have to be very mindful practicing this drill. You and your partners should agree that you'll go at 20-30% speed and always have a "safe word" if you can't tap. In fact the phrase "Tap, tap, tap!" is a great one. The goal is to prevent the submission and escape unscathed.

You can try different versions as well. You might start from different steps within a submission. For example the triangle choke has four steps. Phase 1. The arm goes through and the legs are locked around the neck Phase 2. The hips are raised as the arm goes across Phase 3. Foot goes to the hip as you cut an angle and pull their head into the crook of the knee Phase 4. You grab your shin and lock the legs into the triangle position.

The objective would be to try escaping from different steps. This will help improve your defenses and allow you to identify vulnerable points in the attack sequence. By understanding each phase of the submission you gain a deeper understanding of its mechanics. To deepen your understanding of the move you can begin to strategize your escape and reduce the threats within each step.

For example:

Triangle choke from guard Phase One -

As they attempt to push your arm through you can pull both arms through (double under-hooks position). You can also work on improving your posture by elevating your head on step one. I call this the "Jack-in-the-box." Your goal is to immediately pop up your head when they push your arm through the legs.

Triangle choke Phase Two -

As they attempt to bring your arm across you can try to step your same side leg over their body to escape. You can also try to elevate your head and make posture. As you do this you can pull your arm through and out of the lock (the arm they are trying to bring across).

Triangle Choke Phase Three -

As they try to cut an angle you can square up your shoulders to nullify the movement.

Triangle Choke Phase Four -

You're now in a fully locked triangle choke. Like in the "Hunger Games", May the odds be forever in your favor. (Probably not likely though) It is possible to escape in stage four, but it is very difficult. With a triangle choke your emphasis should be on making sure you can breathe. Even if it means creating just enough space to get some air. Always be extra careful with escaping submissions at steps 3-4.

Here are more examples of the steps that accompany a technique with the potential defense strategies for each submission:

Armbar from the mount steps -

Reach across with your right arm and lift up their right shoulder.

Slide your left knee into the space (near their head) where the shoulder was while simultaneously posting your right leg.

Push down on their head with your left hand and slide your left leg over their head.

As you fall back pinch your knees together as you elevate your hips skyward.

(That describes a basic mount armbar, details can vary)

Armbar counter defense at each phase -

- As they attempt to elevate your shoulder you pin it to the floor by keeping your elbows attached to your chest. In other words, don't leave any space from the point of your elbows and your own body. The tips should be buried into your torso. This makes it nearly impossible to elevate your shoulders. You can also bump your hips every time they grab your arms. Attempt to bump them to the corners (sides of your body). This will force them to base on the floor (not get face planted) and it disrupts their base (gets them off balance).

- As they lift up your shoulder to slide their knee in place of it - place your left hand into the back of their right leg which is now posting up. Turn your hips towards them and get up before they can slide their left leg over your head. For gi training you can also grab your right side lapel with your right arm to protect it while escaping.

- As they attempt to bring their leg over your head you will connect your right hand to your left bicep (much like an RNC position). This will protect your arm and allow you to push their leg off from your head with your left arm. Without the leg covering your head, you can escape. The key is that you cannot let your right arm (the one they're arm-barring) be extended straight (parallel to their body). You can also focus on getting your right elbow away from their pelvic bone (the fulcrum) and to the floor. When your elbow is on the floor (below the fulcrum) they cannot apply an armbar.

Phase four of any submission is always the most difficult to escape. This is particularly true of the armbar where the risk is high and the reward of escaping is low. When your partner has your arm under control and you're not grabbing onto anything this is called an "open chain." When your hands are locked together or when you're grabbing your own gi, this is referred to as a "closed chain." Escaping with an open chain is risky at best. There's an escape technique known as "the hitchhiker," where you turn your thumb away from your partner to maneuver your arm out of a straight arm-bar. **Be very careful practicing this escape as you can turn incorrectly and be injured.**

We have shared two versions of escape strategies from each step within the attack. You can continue exploring this drill with other techniques and submissions.

Takedown belly down takedown -

This is a drill where you can explore your takedown defense along with attack strategies. Here's how it works. Decide ahead of time who will do the initial takedown. Move around with your partner and they will attempt different takedowns at a moderate speed. You can defend the first few, but let them hit the third or fourth attempt. As they penetrate into the takedown your job is to defend it by going belly down into a sprawl position. You then immediately follow up with your own takedown which they don't defend. When you return to your feet you reverse the roles (you do the takedown and they defend).

Creative mindset - Recognizing the importance of developing a strong mind-set around your grappling is crucial to your long-term success.

Maintaining laser point focus during grappling cultivates a disciplined mental state that permeates through all aspects of your training.

As a beginner its very easy to get sucked into a cyclone of "fight or flight." Conversely as a more seasoned practitioner you can often get lazy with your thinking and lose focus. You shouldn't be reacting from fear any more than you should be dismissive of your opponents attacks.

There's a lot of value in utilizing muscle memory during your rolls. It frees the mind and allows you to focus on other aspects of your game. If you're trying to apply an armbar but have to think through every single step, it will be very hard to put attention elsewhere. The four main steps will require all of your conscious effort. But if you had developed muscle memory around the armbar you could focus on preparing for potential counters and defenses.

The downside of muscle memory is you are often locked into habitual patterns with little time to switch gears when needed. Muscle memory can be very effective but can also be a 'double-edged sword.' Therefore it's important to play 'brain games' during your grappling sessions to keep your mind alert and adaptive.

"Telling a Story" drill - (done while grappling)

In this drill you will purposely try and mentally 'grapple and chew gum' at the same time. Start by closing your eyes and use your minds eye to picture yourself in a park on an early morning. Imagine that you're walking down a trail. You want to create an elaborate mental experience while you're grappling. Imagine details of everything you are seeing and experiencing. The objective is to distract and divide your attention between the physical act of grappling and the detailed mental imagery of your story. Essentially you're mental multi-tasking, switching between the high intensity physical act of grappling and an immersive mental narrative.

Drill set up:

Decide who will be the **Mental Imaginer (MI)** and who will be the **Active Attacker (AA)**. Throughout the round the **AA** will keep the action going while the **MI** will be engaging in defensive counter attacks.

Visualization:

The MI will use their mind's eye to create an elaborate, detailed story of their walk in the woods. Go into intricate details about the weather, sites you see and senses that are engaged. (Sight smells, hearing, taste, touch, interactions, etc.)

Continuous grappling:

While you're visualizing keep grappling and maintain your uninterrupted focus.

Switch roles:

After an agreed upon time switch the roles of the AA and MI.

Discussion:

At the end of both rounds share your detailed story along with what physically occurred during the round.

Objective:

To mentally multi-task which enhances cognitive load under unpredictable circumstances. Over time practitioners will be able to maintain better focus while adapting to unpredictable circumstances.

"Allegory of the Cave" drill -

In this mental exercise you will close your eyes during the round and imagine yourself in a dark cave. The "cave" drill is a mental visualization technique that merges the principles of Plato's "Allegory of the Cave" with the tactile reality of grappling. The goal is to try and mentally "see" each counter move as it happens in real time. As you see yourself moving though a dark cave an image appears before your eyes of each move that you should take as your partner attacks.

The goal is to train your mind to analyze and predict responses to moves based solely on touch, instinct and mental imagery.

Drill set up:

Be sure to explain the drill to your partner in advance and prepare to switch roles when needed. Decide in advance who will be the MI and who will be the AA.

MI - Start the round by seeing yourself standing in front of a cave entrance. In front of you is absolute darkness. Behind you is light. As the round begins you will see yourself moving forward into complete darkness. In front of you images will appear as you begin to initiate touch with your partner.

AA - Move at a slow, controlled pace that allows your partner time to respond. (Start at 10-15% speed)

MI - In complete darkness imagine a luminescent light that briefly reveals an image of each counter move as it happens. This image is your guide. Eventually you will become quicker and more proficient in your response, eliminating the lag time of conscious thought.

AA - Over time increase the "intensity variation." Start the round at 10-15% effort and speed while gradually increasing it. This will expand the boundaries of your mental acuity.

Distraction integration:

As you progress with the drill begin to add external noises and loud music. This is excellent for competitors who want to improve their tournament focus.

The cave drill is an excellent test of mental fortitude and and tactile awareness. Just like the prisoner's in Plato's allegory who move from the ignorance of the dark cave to the enlightened reality outside. This drill aims to take practitioners away from mere physical reactions to a heightened mental awareness and intuitive understanding.

"Blind-folded multi-partner drill" -

You can also introduce the added element of multiple partners. In this drill, you will grapple with your eyes closed, and throughout the round, new partners will rotate in. You will keep your eyes shut, so you won't know whom you're grappling with.

Drill set up:

Have the group surround one person who is in the middle with their eyes closed.

Each person will be given a number and then the circle will be scrambled so the person in the middle cannot recognize their partners.

One person will call out the numbers and the corresponding person will grapple the individual in the center. The person in the center stays in for the entire round. When a number is called go right to the center and begin grappling from whatever position you're in. (Avoid slapping and bumping, just grapple)

Objective:

The goal is to develop your proprioception (limb awareness) while focusing on your partners strength, movements and strategy. Maintain a relaxed calm approach so you don't miss any opportunities. This drill will also help you adapt to the ever-changing energy exchange that each new partner brings. It also allows you to 'let go' of preconceived notions of attaching skill levels and belt ranks to individuals. When you don't know who you are rolling with, you are free from further mental constraints.

Mission:

With this operation the mission is to explore and build your creative instincts. I've often heard practitioners say, "I don't have a creative bone in my body!" That's fine because the framework of BJJ is such that it allows for seamless integration of creativity. You can often adapt and create on the fly if you're open to it.

Remember a closed mind will only get you so far, but an open one can take you to new heights. The beauty of BJJ lies in its fluidity and adaptability, making it an ideal platform for nurturing creativity.

Every practitioner has the potential to develop this skill through practice and exploration. Remember, creativity in BJJ is not about reinventing the wheel, but rather about seeing the myriad of possibilities within the existing framework.

You can further cultivate your creative instincts in BJJ by observing and learning from others. Watch how upper belts adapt their style and strategies in different situations. Experiment with new techniques during grappling sessions, and don't be afraid to make mistakes. These are opportunities for learning and growth.

Creativity is a muscle that strengthens with use. Utilize the drills that we've included in this operation to build your creative impulse. Incorporate them into your regular grappling sessions to enhance your ability to think creatively on the mats.

These exercises are designed not just to improve your physical skills but also to encourage mental flexibility and innovation in your approach to BJJ. Don't worry about making mistakes while drilling. Focus on the process and not perfection!

Debriefing Assessment:

Review your ongoing journey as to black belt and beyond. Are you continuing to challenge yourself both on and off the mats? Reflect on your contributions to the BJJ community and personal growth. Have you embraced opportunities to innovate and lead within your sphere of influence?

Pinpoint areas for personal and community growth. Consider developing new teaching methods, exploring uncharted techniques, or enhancing your academy's culture. How can you better foster a supportive environment for all practitioners?

Utilize feedback from students, peers, and self-assessment to guide your developmental path. Are there new needs or desires within the community that you can address? Reflect on how your leadership can evolve to meet these challenges.

Outline your legacy goals for the next year and beyond. Plan specific initiatives, such as mentorship programs, seminars, or collaborative projects, to enrich your community's experience and your personal mastery of BJJ.

PART IV:
CONTINUING THE JOURNEY

Reinforcements for Veterans

Jiu-Jitsu has the ability to help us in so many ways, but sometimes we might need some extra back up. For my fellow veterans these are some great resources… and ***thank you for your service!***

Remember, asking for help when you need it shows strength.

Get social and share your story and hear those of others online.

Involve loved ones in your choices. This will give you support and perspective in your decision making.

Consider having a trusted source to openly communicate what you went through and what still surfaces.

Veterans PTSD nationwide

https://www.ptsd.va.gov/gethelp/tx_programs.asp

Veterans crisis hotline

https://www.veteranscrisisline.net/

Veterans substance abuse help

https://www.mentalhealth.va.gov/substance-use/index.asp?utm_
source=google&utm_medium=cpc&utm_campaign=search_va_
sud_gen&utm_term=phrase-match&utm_content=help%20for%20
addiction&gclid=EAIaIQobChMIhuKkn5T0hAMVqBWtBh1lzQAsE-
AAYAiAAEgLd5_D_BwE

Mission:

Civilians - thank a Veteran for their service.

Veterans - again thank you, blessings and take good care of yourself.

Giving to the Future

What does it truly mean to leave a lasting impact in BJJ? As we advance in our training, the focus often shifts from personal achievement to fostering growth and enrichment within the community.

BJJ isn't merely about the medals and titles; it's about the knowledge shared, the lives touched, and the culture nurtured within your sphere of influence. It's about planting seeds that will grow long after you've left the mat. Reflect on what aspects of your BJJ you find most fulfilling and envision how these elements can be passed on to others.

Contribution can take many forms—from coaching and teaching to simply being a positive presence in your gym. Engage in discussions, share your story, and be open to learning from others, too. Every conversation, every roll, is an opportunity to strengthen the bonds within your BJJ family.

Mentorship might be just what you've been missing. It's not just about teaching techniques; it's about guiding younger practitioners through the ups and downs of their practice. Share your insights on dealing with losses, managing injuries, and balancing life with training. Remember, a good mentor doesn't create followers; they nurture future leaders.

To leave a lasting impact, be intentional in your actions and words. Develop a personal philosophy that reflects your values and make it a cornerstone of your interactions. Consider how you handle both victories and defeats, and how you treat your training partners. These elements are as contagious as they are influential.

Mission:

Giving to the future of BJJ goes beyond the mat. It is about creating a positive ripple effect that will continue to inspire and influence long after your direct involvement. By focusing on community, mentorship, and lasting impact, you are not just a participant in the sport but a pivotal architect of its future. Let your legacy be defined not just by what you achieved, but by how you uplifted others along the way.

Community and Support Networks in BJJ

Our tribes are strong communities that can transform the BJJ experience, providing not only a place to learn but also a source of motivation and friendship. The right vibe is vital in maintaining enthusiasm and commitment to the sport. Let's delve into the psychological and physical benefits of being part of a BJJ community, such as reduced feelings of isolation, increased encouragement, and improved mental health.

Being part of BJJ offers numerous benefits, particularly for those over 40:

- Engaging with like-minded individuals helps combat loneliness, fostering a sense of belonging.

- Training with peers provides accountability and excitement, helping you stay committed to your goals.

- The camaraderie and support of a community can alleviate stress and anxiety, contributing to overall well-being and improving your mental health.

Inclusivity is essential for a thriving BJJ community. This means creating environments where all feel welcome, regardless of age, skill level or physical capability.

Here's how we can foster inclusivity:

- Adjust your Learning Methods and Class Structures: Tailor classes to meet any needs. This might include modified warm-ups, lower-intensity drills, and techniques that are easier on the joints.

- Ensuring Respectful Communication: Promote a culture of respect and kindness. Address unconscious biases and encourage open dialogue.

- Find Flexible Training Options: Seek various class times and formats to accommodate different schedules and lifestyles.

Building connections among practitioners involves more than just regular training sessions. Consider these activities to strengthen bonds within your community:

- Attend gatherings outside of training, such as group dinners, movie nights, or outdoor activities. These events let us connect on a personal level.

- Try a Seminar or Workshop. Look for local legends or support a guest instructor rolling into town.

- Get the buddy system going. Experienced practitioners find a newcomer and vice versa. Mentors can share their knowledge and experiences, helping newcomers integrate into the community more smoothly.

- Technology can play a crucial role in strengthening community ties:

- Utilize online platforms through social media and join groups to stay engaged, share educational content, and facilitate discussions outside the gym.

- Take a virtual training session. If you may not always be able to attend in person try an online class or tutorial. This is a fun way to connect with everyone involved worldwide.

Mission:

Build a supportive BJJ community for yourself through physical and virtual resources.

Understand the exact essentials for sustaining your active participation in the sport. This means making sure you know what's important to you to receive from your investment? Do you want like minded individuals or characters that challenge the regular script? Find what works for your style so you'll be sure to stick around.

Survival Experts: JOE & DEAN from XMARTIAL

Joe - Owner - White belt level with a couple of years experience in BJJ but mixed with Muay Thai

Dean - Athlete manager - Very new to Jiu-Jitsu, a couple of months training

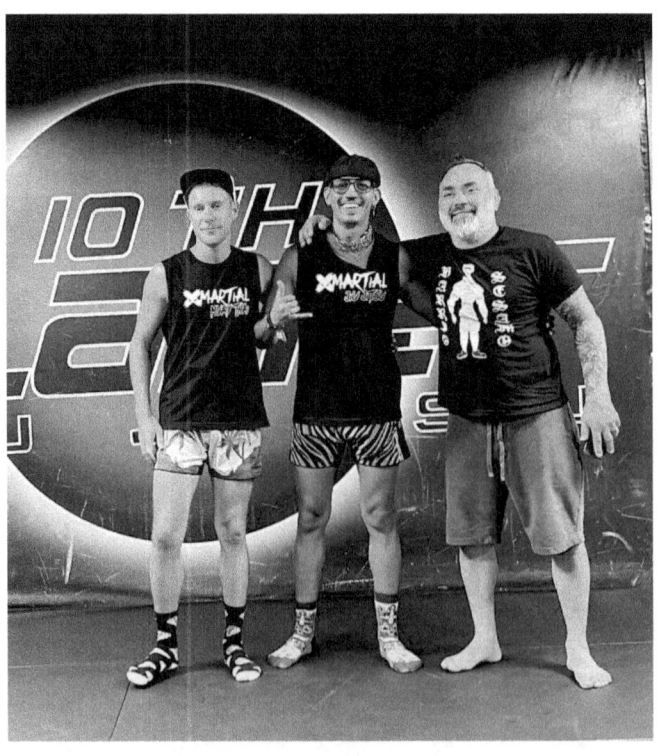

Intel:

I have had a dream for sometime to create a line of training gear with designs for the over 40 athlete. I came across the very popular Xmartial brand and was quickly blown away by the number of designs they offered!

We are excited for our collaboration with this great company that offers high quality products with beautiful designs. This collection features BJJAfter40 designs, each adorned with cool sayings that resonate with our experiences and the journey we embrace in Brazilian Jiu-Jitsu. The awesome designs reflect the spirit and passion of our over 40 community, offering both style and functionality on the mats. Xmartial is also known for giving back to the BJJ community through its sponsorship initiative to empower young athletes in underserved communities.

From the Source:

Right now we are promoting the Dojo Roadshow, our Jiu-Jitsu based show on YouTube where we travel across the US in an RV to visit gyms, competitions and meet the who's who of the sport. We are sponsoring athletes along the way.

We sponsor athletes of all ages and all levels, and in 2023 alone we gave away over $50,000 of gear.

We also have a gym partnership program that helps gyms with products, provides free gear to their coaches and helps them obtain new students via our social media and email promotion.

We have also just launched an initiative where we sponsor kids who are financially unable to train. We set them up with gear and pay the first few months membership for them in order to give them a start in martial arts.

In terms of the culture for over 40s, we see it thriving as more and more tournaments offer a masters division. Also amazing communities like BJJ after 40 help massively to get people involved.

If BJJ were a superhero, the power that it has given us is the power to be able to work remotely, travel and to help people in the community (that is more specifically to the business that we run) but on a personal level it helps with becoming more social with people.

As someone under 40, only just haha, I would say that practitioners over 40 give me a lot of confidence and make me realize that it is never too late to get involved in this amazing sport. And in terms of what the youth can learn from the over 40 community, I would say patience.

Everyone wants things to come super fast but the Jiu-Jitsu journey is a marathon, not a sprint.

Workout and Nutrition Plans

Navigating through the complex world of fitness and nutrition can be daunting. Let's explore the essentials to brining your training to the kitchen and gym.

Dynamic Preparation and Recovery

Every session on the mats should begin with a purposeful warm-up and end with a thorough cool-down—these are your bookends of protection. Warm-ups should activate your muscles through dynamic movements that mimic the actions of BJJ, preparing your body for the explosive demands of grappling. Cool-downs should involve gentle stretching and flexibility exercises to ease the muscles back into a state of rest, promoting faster recovery and reducing the risk of injury.

Strength and Sustainability

Strength training is not just about lifting weights; it's about constructing a fortress around your joints, supporting bone density, and enhancing muscle endurance. Incorporate exercises that strengthen the core, improve joint stability, and support overall body strength without overloading your frame. Emphasize functional movements that translate directly to improved performance on the mats.

Mobility Matters

Flexibility and mobility are your secret weapons for maintaining a wide range of motion and preventing injuries. Regular mobility exercises help keep your joints supple and can significantly improve your grappling technique by allowing for deeper, more controlled movements.

Cardiovascular Care

Low-impact cardio options such as swimming, cycling, or even brisk walking are essential to maintain cardiovascular health without stressing your joints. These activities help manage weight, improve heart health, and increase stamina—allowing you to train longer and recover faster.

Nutritional Tactics

Adjust your macronutrient ratios to fuel your body efficiently. High-quality proteins are crucial for muscle repair, especially after intense training sessions. Carbohydrates should be aligned with your activity levels—higher on training days and moderated on rest days. Healthy fats are vital for long-term energy and supporting overall health.

Incorporate anti-inflammatory foods like turmeric, berries, and fatty fish into your diet to help reduce recovery times and combat age-related inflammation. Remember, the key to effective nutrition is consistency and variety.

Hydration and Supplements

Hydration is the cornerstone of peak athletic performance. Tailor your hydration needs based on your sweat rate and the intensity of your training. Don't overlook the importance of electrolytes that help maintain fluid balance and prevent cramping.

Supplements like omega-3 fatty acids, vitamin D, and protein powders can support recovery, while joint health supplements such as glucosamine may offer additional benefits for older athletes.

Mission:

Create a Structured Plan: Begin by assessing your current fitness level and nutritional habits. Design a workout schedule that includes strength, flexibility, and cardio, while tailoring your diet to support your energy needs and recovery.

Incorporate Variety: Keep your body guessing and your mind engaged by varying your workouts and trying new recipes that align with your nutritional goals.

Monitor and Adapt: Regularly review your progress and be ready to adapt your plans as you evolve. What works today may need adjustment tomorrow as you grow stronger and more skilled.

Seek Expert Advice: Consult with your coach and fitness experts who understand the unique needs of aging athletes. Their guidance can be invaluable in fine-tuning your plan to your specific requirements.

By embracing these strategies, you ensure that your Brazilian Jiu-Jitsu is not just about survival, but about thriving. With the right plan in place, you can look forward to many more years of rolling, learning, and growing. Let's get started and roll towards a healthier, stronger you!

Glossary

Active Stabilizers vs. Inert Stabilizers:

- **Active Stabilizers:** Muscles that actively control the position of joints.

- **Inert Stabilizers:** Muscles that do not actively control joint positions but contribute to joint stability passively.

These concepts are essential for maintaining balance and stability in various positions, enabling more effective control and submission execution.

Aerodynamics: The study of the properties of moving air and how objects move through such air. In BJJ, it refers metaphorically to the fluidity of movement. Understanding aerodynamics can help practitioners move more smoothly and efficiently, reducing resistance from both the air and opponents.

Angular Momentum (L = mvr): In physics, angular momentum refers to the quantity of rotation of a body, which is the product of its moment of inertia and its angular velocity. Angular momentum is crucial in executing sweeps and spins. Understanding this helps a practitioner maintain balance while rotating their body or an opponent's, enhancing the effectiveness of maneuvers.

Debriefing: In a BJJ context, a reflective discussion after a training session or event where participants review what was learned, discuss the effectiveness of techniques, and plan future training strategies.

Defense Frame Work: This the counter / reversal side of a submission. What is the one thing that allows the move to work? A triangle for example, relies on one arm to be extended inside your partners legs and one arm retracted. Without this framework a triangle will not work. Another example would be the armbar. It cannot work unless the elbow joint is above the fulcrum, not below it. Discovering and locating the DF will allow you to effectively counter any submission technique. By utilizing this concept you can defend moves without understanding every detail of the moves execution.

DTP: Demonstrate. Teach. Perform.

Dynamic Loads: These involve forces that change over time, like those experienced during a sweep. Knowing the difference helps a practitioner apply the right kind of force during training or competition to maintain control or execute movements efficiently.

Fluid Dynamics: The study of how fluids (liquids and gases) move and interact with objects. Analogous to how practitioners should "flow" around resistance, utilizing the path of least resistance to conserve energy and maintain positional advantage.

Force Distribution: The way force is spread over an area. In BJJ, this often refers to how a practitioner applies their weight across different parts of an opponent's body. Effective force distribution in positions like side control can increase control over an opponent and reduce their ability to escape.

Head Positioning: involves controlling the orientation of the head in relation to the spine and the rest of the body.

Leverage: Using the mechanical advantage gained by the use of a lever, which in BJJ translates to using one's limbs to create a pivotal point that maximizes the force applied to an opponent.

LTT: Leverage, Timing, Technique.

- **Leverage:** includes the use of classical Newtonian physics, active / inert stabilizers, force distribution , static and dynamic loads, angular momentum, etc.

- **Timing:** using predictive responses to force your partner to respond in your favor.

- **Technique:** is made of the four primary steps of a move, the "secret sauce", and the defensive framework.

Mission: In this guide, a mission refers to a specific goal or task within the broader scope of BJJ training, emphasizing strategic approaches similar to military operations.

Neuroplasticity: The brain's ability to reorganize itself by forming new neural connections throughout life. In BJJ, this refers to the way practitioners can continually learn and adapt their skills through repetitive practice and strategic thinking.

Operations: Structured training sequences in the guide, each designed to achieve specific learning outcomes in BJJ, analogous to military operations which are coordinated efforts to achieve a decisive goal.

QR Code (Quick Response Code): A type of matrix barcode that contains information about the item to which it is attached, used in this guide to link to multimedia learning tools such as technique videos and audio meditations.

Secret Sauce: the aspect of the move that makes it more efficient, reliable and effective. Often called the "magic of the move." The move can still work without the secret sauce - however you'll need to use a physical attributes (martial) in its absence.

Spinal Alignment: Refers to the proper positioning of the spine to maintain an optimal balance of forces across the vertebrae and discs.

Static vs. Dynamic Loads:

- **Static Loads:** These are forces applied slowly or are constant, like maintaining pressure in side control.

- **Dynamic Loads:** Force and pressure that moves from one spot to another .

Tactical Maneuvers: In BJJ, these are planned movements and techniques designed to achieve an advantage over an opponent, akin to military strategies used in combat scenarios.

Technique: this is your four primary steps of a technique. If you were to distill any move down to four steps, what would they be? When you execute a move you cannot advance forward in the technique without successfully completing the previous step.

Vestibular System: located in the inner ear, is crucial for balance and spatial orientation. It helps the brain process changes in head movement relative to gravity.

Contact Information

It was such an honor to have everyone's helping hands create this book.

We highly encourage you to show your support to the Survival Experts! Scan the QR code below and find tons more online content from our contributors.

Subscribe to the Survival Experts YouTube Playlist Page
https:///www.youtube.com/playlist?list=PLwb5iQup993_kWP8jXM_
jueeY6kzd19Wb

Ari Knazan

https://enterchaos.com/,
https://submissions101.com/

Bong Abad

website: www.gawakoto.com
Instagram: @gawakoto
Facebook: facebook.com/gawakoto

Brent Burniston

www.Subconsciousbjj.com @Subconsciousbjj- IG
www.SJJAssociation.com

Garry Parrett

Email: ozman26_@hotmail.com
Phone: (715) 927-0767

Marco Lala

Website: fightingsecrets.com
YouTube: https://youtube.com/@tettsubushi
Email: fightingsecretsonline@gmail.com

Marty Josey

Websites: https://www.theintentionalchill.com
https://www.amazon.com/See-You-Mat-Perspective-Transformation/dp/
B08KH3VMKY

Mark "Funk" Roberts

Kettlebell for Fighters -
https://kettlebellspartanacademy.com/kettlebell-mma-workouts
Facebook- facebook.com/FunkMMA
IG-@funkrobertsfitness

Mike Jolly

https://www.iron-neck.com/

Ryan Ford

Instagram: @GringoRyan

Vlad Koulikov

Instagram: https://instagram.com/sambo_fusion
igshid=MjEwN2IyYWYwYw==

Website: http://sambofusion.com/blog/119066/Curriculum
Phone: (845)-421-8809

XMartial

https://www.xmartial.com/
*Use Code BJJAFTER40 for 10% off!

www.ingramcontent.com/pod-product-compliance
Lightning Source LLC
Chambersburg PA
CBHW060853120626
46553CB00001B/73